RENAL DIET COOKBOOK FOR BEGINNERS

THE ULTIMATE GUIDE WITH 149 LOW SODIUM, POTASSIUM, AND PHOSPHORUS RECIPES. A QUICK, EASY AND TASTY FORMULA TO FACE EARLY STAGE OF KIDNEY DISEASE AND AVOID DIALYSIS

Elizabeth Meylight

Table of Contents

Introduction

The Renal Diet Cookbook is intended to help those people suffering from kidney disease to live kidney stone-free lives. Liberating oneself from the kidney stone dilemma is not a fate worse than death. It's quite liberating to live life without the fear of kidney stones lurking about.

Renal diets may be divided into two broad categories: The strict diet and the liberal diet. The strict diet is the traditional higher protein, lower phosphorus diet typically recommended to patients suffering from kidney disease. The liberal diet is low protein, low phosphorus, and the reason for the latter is due to the fact that the blood phosphorus levels are closely regulated with liberal diets, hence the need for much closer monitoring.

Whether you are to be judged as a strict dieter or liberal dieter is your own decision. Each person is different, so the goal for each person will be different

About the Diet:

You may not realize, but your kidneys are the most important organs in your body. Everyone has two kidneys, one on his right side and the other on the left. These internal organs are about the size of your fist. They weigh about 1 pound. The kidneys have many important functions. They regulate fluid balance, filter wastes, including dissolved proteins and excess minerals from the body, and help rid the blood of extra red blood cells, which decreases blood thickness. Diets that are high in protein can damage your kidneys. The kidneys excrete waste products into the urine. Some waste products are dangerous; however, your kidneys can remove many of them. In fact, they can remove even more wastes than are present. If the wastes are not removed, they build up in the body and do damage. The renal diet aims not at weight loss but ANTISEPTIC CLEANSING, which is absolutely safe and helps you feel very fresh and lighter.

What to Eat and What to Avoid in the Renal Diet

Many foods work well within the renal diet. Once you see the available variety, it will not seem as restrictive or difficult to follow. The key is to focus on foods with a high level of nutrients, which make it easier for the kidneys to process the waste by not adding too much that the body needs to discard. Balance is a major factor in maintaining and improving long-term renal function.

• **Garlic**: An excellent, vitamin-rich food for the immune system, garlic is a tasty substitute for salt in a variety of dishes. It acts as a significant source of vitamin C and B6 while aiding the kidneys in ridding the body of unwanted toxins. It's a great and healthy way to add flavor to skillet meals, pasta, soups, and stews.

• **Berries**: All berries are considered a good renal diet food due to their high level of fiber, antioxidants, and delicious taste, making them an easy option to include as a light snack or as an ingredient in smoothies, salads, and light desserts. Just one handful of blueberries can provide almost one day's vitamin C requirement, as well as a boost of fiber, which is good for weight loss and maintenance.

• **Bell peppers**: Flavorful and easy to enjoy both raw and cooked; bell peppers offer a good vitamin C source, vitamin A, and fiber. Along with other kidney-friendly foods, they make the detoxification process much easier while boosting your body's nutrient level to prevent further health conditions and reduce existing deficiencies.

• **Onions**: This nutritious and tasty vegetable is excellent as a companion to garlic in many dishes or on its own. Like garlic, onions can provide flavor as an alternative to salt and provide a good source of vitamin C, vitamin B, manganese, and fiber, as well. Adding just one quarter or half of the onion is often enough for most meals because of its strong and pungent flavor.

• **Macadamia nuts**: If you enjoy nuts and seeds as snacks, you may learn that many contain high amounts of phosphorus and should be avoided or limited as much as possible. Fortunately, macadamia nuts are an easier option to digest and process, as they contain much lower amounts of phosphorus and make an excellent substitute for other nuts. They are a good source of other nutrients, as well, such as vitamin B, copper, manganese, iron, and healthy fats.

• **Pineapple**: Unlike other fruits that are high in potassium, pineapple is an option that can be enjoyed more often than bananas and kiwis. Citrus fruits are generally high in potassium as well, so if you find yourself craving an orange or grapefruit, choose pineapple instead. In addition to providing high levels of vitamin B and fiber, pineapples can reduce inflammation thanks to an enzyme called bromelain.

• **Mushrooms**: In general, mushrooms are a safe and healthy option for the renal diet, especially the shiitake variety, high in nutrients such as selenium, vitamin B, and manganese. They contain a moderate amount of plant-based protein, which is easier for your body to digest and use than animal proteins. Shiitake and portobello mushrooms are often used in vegan diets as a meat substitute due to their texture and pleasant flavor.

Foods to Avoid

Eating restrictions might be different depending upon your level of kidney disease. If you are in the early stages of kidney disease, you may have different restrictions compared to those in the end-stage of renal disease or kidney failure. In contrast to this, people with an end-stage renal disease requiring dialysis will face different eating restrictions. Let's discuss some of the foods to avoid while being on the renal diet.

Dark-Colored Colas contain calories, sugar, phosphorus, etc. They contain phosphorus to enhance flavor, increase its life, and avoid discoloration, which can be found in a product's ingredient list. This addition of phosphorus varies depending on the type of cola. Mostly, the dark-colored colas contain 50–100 mg in a 200-ml serving. Therefore, dark colas should be avoided on a renal diet.

Avocados are a source of many nutritious characteristics, plus their strong fats, fiber, and antioxidants. Individuals suffering from kidney disease should avoid them because they are rich in potassium. 150 grams of an avocado provides a whopping 727 mg of potassium. Therefore, avocados, including guacamole, must be avoided on a renal diet, especially if you are on parole to watch your potassium intake.

Canned foods, including soups, vegetables, and beans, are low in cost but contain high amounts of sodium due to the addition of salt to increase its life. Due to this amount of sodium inclusion in canned goods, it is better for people with kidney disease should avoid consumption. Opt for lower-sodium content with the label "no salt added." One more way is to drain or rinse canned foods, such as canned beans and tuna, which could decrease the sodium content by 33–80%, depending on the product.

Brown rice is a whole grain containing a higher concentration of potassium and phosphorus than its white rice counterpart. One cup of already cooked brown rice possesses about 150 mg of phosphorus and 154 mg of potassium, whereas one cup of already cooked white rice has about 69 mg of phosphorus and 54 mg of potassium. Bulgur, buckwheat, pearled barley, and couscous are equally beneficial, low-phosphorus options and might be a good alternative instead of brown rice.

Bananas are high potassium content, low in sodium, and provide 422 mg of potassium per banana. It might disturb your daily balanced potassium intake to 2,000 mg if a banana is a daily staple.

Whole-Wheat bread may harm individuals with kidney disease. But for healthy individuals, it is recommended over refined, white flour bread. White bread is recommended instead of whole-wheat varieties for individuals with kidney disease just because it has phosphorus and potassium. If you add more bran and whole grains to the bread, then the amount of phosphorus and potassium contents goes higher.

Oranges and orange juice are enriched with vitamin C content and potassium. 184 grams provide 333 mg of potassium and 473 mg of potassium in one cup of orange juice. With these calculations, they must be avoided or used in a limited amount while being on a renal diet. Other alternatives for oranges and orange juice are apples, grapes, and their cinder or juices as they possess low potassium contents.

Potatoes and sweet potatoes, which are potassium-rich vegetables with 156g containing 610 mg of potassium, whereas 114 g contain 541 mg of potassium, which is relatively high. Some of the high- potassium foods, likewise potatoes and sweet potatoes, could also be soaked or leached to lessen the concentration of potassium contents. Cut them into small and thin pieces and boil those for at least 10 minutes can reduce the potassium content by about 50%. Potatoes that are soaked in a wide pot of water for as low as four hours before cooking could possess even less potassium content than those not soaked before cooking. This is known as "potassium leaching" or the "double cook Direction."

Snack foods like pretzels, chips, and crackers are foods that lack nutrients and are much higher in salt. It is very easy to take above the suggested portion, which leads to an even greater salt intake than planned. If chips, being made from potatoes, they will contain a significant amount of potassium as well.

If you are suffering or living with kidney disease, reducing your potassium, phosphorus, and sodium intake is an essential aspect for managing and tackling the disease. The foods with high-potassium, high-sodium, and high-phosphorus content listed above should always be limited or avoided. These restrictions and nutrients intakes may differ depending on the level of damage to your kidneys. Following a renal diet might be a daunting procedure and a restrictive one most of the time. But, working with your physician and nutrition specialist and a renal dietitian can assist you to formulate a renal diet specific to your individual needs.

Breakfast

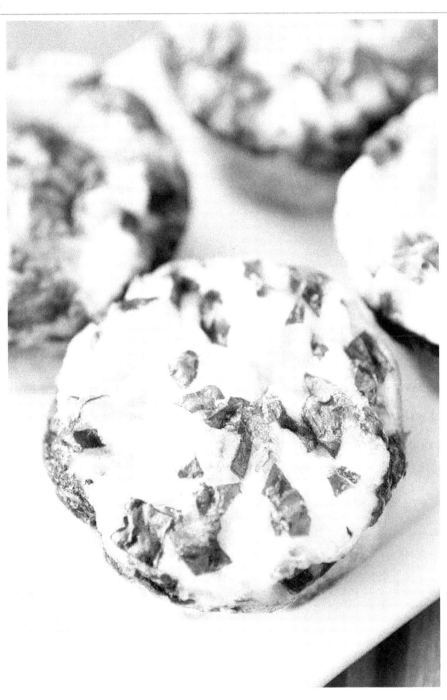

Chicken Egg Rolls

Preparation time: 10 minutes

Cooking time: 12 minutes

Servings: 14

Ingredients:

- 1 lb. cooked chicken, diced
- 1/2 lb. bean sprouts
- 1/2 lb. cabbage, shredded
- 1 cup onion, chopped
- 2 tablespoons olive oil
- 1 tablespoon low sodium soy sauce
- 1 clove of garlic, minced
- 20 egg roll wrappers
- Oil for frying

Directions:

1. Add everything to a suitable bowl except for the roll wrappers.
2. Mix these ingredients well to prepare the filling, then marinate for 30 minutes.
3. Place the roll wrappers on the working surface and divide the prepared filling on them.
4. Fold the roll wrappers as per the package instructions and keep them aside.
5. Add oil to a deep wok and heat it to 350° F.
6. Deep the egg rolls until golden brown on all sides.
7. Transfer the egg rolls to a plate lined with a paper towel to absorb all the excess oil.
8. Serve warm.

Nutrition:

- Calories: 212
- Total Fat: 3.8g
- Cholesterol: 29mg
- Sodium: 150mg
- Carbohydrates: 29g
- Sugar: 0.9g
- Protein: 14.9g
- Phosphorus: 93 mg
- Potassium: 171mg

Salmon Bagel Toast

Preparation time: 10 minutes

Cooking time: 5 minutes

Servings: 2

Ingredients:

- 1 plain bagel, cut in half
- 2 tablespoons cream cheese
- 1/3 cup English cucumber, thinly sliced
- 3 oz. smoked salmon, sliced
- 3 rings red onion
- 1/2 teaspoon capers, drained

Directions:

1. Toast each half of the bagel in a skillet until golden brown.
2. Cover one of the toasted halves with cream cheese.
3. Set the cucumber, salmon, onion and capers on top of each bagel half.
4. Enjoy.

Nutrition:

- Calories: 223
- Total Fat: 6.2g
- Saturated Fat: 2.8g
- Cholesterol: 21mg
- Sodium: 185mg
- Carbohydrates: 27.5g
- Dietary Fiber: 1.3g
- Sugar: 3g
- Protein: 13.9g
- Calcium: 62mg
- Phosphorus: 79mg
- Potassium: 151mg

Cinnamon Toast Strata

Preparation time: 10 minutes

Cooking time: 50 minutes

Servings: 12

Ingredients:

- 1 lb. loaf cinnamon raisin bread, cubed
- 8 oz. package cream cheese, diced
- 1 cup apples, peeled and diced
- 8 eggs
- 2 1/2 cups half-and-half cream
- 6 tablespoons butter, melted
- 1/4 cup maple syrup

Directions:

1. Layer a 9x13 inch baking dish with cooking spray.

2. Place 1/2 of the bread cubes in the greased baking dish.

3. Cover the bread cubes with cream cheese, apples, and the other half of the bread.

4. Beat the eggs with the melted butter and maple syrup in a bowl.

5. Pour this egg-butter mixture over the bread layer, then refrigerate for 2 hours.

6. Bake this bread-egg casserole for 50 minutes at 325°F.

7. Slice and garnish with pancake syrup.

8. Enjoy.

Nutrition:

- Calories: 276
- Total Fat: 21.4g
- Saturated Fat: 12.4g
- Cholesterol: 165mg
- Sodium: 195mg
- Carbohydrates: 14.5g
- Dietary Fiber: 0.6g
- Sugar: 7.4g
- Protein: 7.5g
- Calcium: 90mg
- Phosphorus: 194 mg
- Potassium: 162mg

Parmesan Zucchini Frittata

Preparation time: 10 minutes

Cooking time: 35 minutes

Servings: 6

Ingredients:

- 1 tablespoon olive oil
- 1 cup yellow onion, sliced
- 3 cups zucchini, chopped
- 1/2 cup Parmesan cheese, grated
- 8 large eggs
- 1/2 teaspoon black pepper
- 1/8 teaspoon paprika
- 3 tablespoons parsley, chopped

Directions:

1. Toss the zucchinis with the onion, parsley, and all other ingredients in a large bowl.

2. Pour this zucchini-garlic mixture in an 11x7 inches pan and spread it evenly.

3. Bake the zucchini casserole for approximately 35 minutes at 350° F.

4. Cut in slices and serve.

Nutrition:

- Calories: 142
- Total Fat: 9.7g
- Saturated Fat: 2.8g
- Cholesterol: 250mg
- Sodium: 123mg
- Carbohydrates: 4.7g
- Dietary Fiber: 1.3g
- Sugar: 2.4g
- Protein: 10.2g
- Calcium: 73mg
- Phosphorus: 149mg
- Potassium: 99mg

Texas Toast Casserole

Preparation time: 10 minutes

Cooking time: 30 minutes

Servings: 10

Ingredients:

- 1/2 cup butter, melted
- 1 cup brown Swerve
- 1 lb. Texas Toast bread, sliced
- 4 large eggs
- 1 1/2 cup oat milk
- 1 tablespoon vanilla extract
- 2 tablespoons Swerve
- 2 teaspoons cinnamon
- Maple syrup for serving

Directions:

1. Layer a 9x13 inches baking pan with cooking spray.
2. Spread the bread slices at the bottom of the prepared pan.
3. Whisk the eggs with the remaining ingredients in a mixer.
4. Pour this mixture over the bread slices evenly.
5. Bake the bread for 30 minutes at 350° F in a preheated oven.
6. Serve.

Nutrition:

- Calories: 332
- Total Fat: 13.7g
- Saturated Fat: 6.9g
- Cholesterol: 102mg
- Sodium: 160mg
- Carbohydrates: 22.6g
- Dietary Fiber: 2g
- Sugar: 6g
- Protein: 7.4g
- Calcium: 143mg
- Phosphorus: 104mg
- Potassium: 74mg

Mozzarella Cheese Omelette

Preparation time: 10 minutes

Cooking time: 5 minutes

Servings: 2

Ingredients:

- 4 eggs, beaten
- 1/4 cup mozzarella cheese, shredded
- 4 tomato slices
- 1/4 tsp Italian seasoning
- 1/4 tsp dried oregano
- Salt

Directions:

1. In a small bowl, whisk eggs with salt.
2. Spray pan with cooking spray and heat over medium heat.
3. Pour egg mixture into the pan and cook over medium heat.
4. Once eggs are set, then, sprinkle oregano and Italian seasoning on top.
5. Arrange tomato slices on top of the omelet and sprinkle with shredded cheese.
6. Cook omelet for 1 minute.
7. Serve and enjoy.

Nutrition:

- Calories: 285
- Fat: 19 g
- Carbohydrates: 4 g
- Sugar: 3 g
- Protein: 25 g
- Cholesterol: 655 mg
- Sodium: 126 mg
- Phosphorous: 108 mg
- Potassium: 192mg

Sun-Dried Tomato Frittata

Preparation time: 10 minutes

Cooking time: 20 minutes

Servings: 8

Ingredients:

- 12 eggs
- 1/2 tsp dried basil
- 1/4 cup parmesan cheese, grated
- 2 cups baby spinach, shredded
- 1/4 cup sun-dried tomatoes, sliced
- Pepper
- Salt

Directions:

1. Preheat the oven to 425° F.

2. In a large bowl, whisk eggs with pepper and salt.

3. Add remaining ingredients and stir to combine.

4. Spray oven-safe pan with cooking spray.

5. Pour egg mixture into the pan and bake for 20 minutes.

6. Slice and serve.

Nutrition:

- Calories: 115
- Fat: 7 g
- Carbohydrates: 1 g
- Sugar: 1 g
- Protein: 10 g
- Cholesterol: 250 mg
- Sodium: 180 mg
- Potassium: 159 mg
- Phosphorous: 143 mg

Italian Breakfast Frittata

Preparation time: 10 minutes

Cooking time: 45 minutes

Servings: 4

Ingredients:

- 2 cups egg whites
- 1/2 cup mozzarella cheese, shredded
- 1 cup cottage cheese, crumbled
- 1/4 cup fresh basil, sliced
- 1/2 cup roasted red peppers, sliced
- Pepper
- Salt

Directions:

1. Preheat the oven to 375° F.

2. Add all ingredients into a large bowl and whisk well to combine.

3. Pour frittata mixture into the baking dish and bake for 45 minutes.

4. Slice and serve.

Nutrition:

- Calories: 131
- Fat: 2 g
- Carbohydrates: 5 g
- Sugar: 2 g
- Protein: 22 g
- Cholesterol: 6 mg
- Sodium: 199mg
- Potassium: 138 mg
- Phosphorous: 143 mg

Sausage Cheese Bake Omelette

Preparation time: 10 minutes

Cooking time: 45 minutes

Servings: 8

Ingredients:

- 16 eggs
- 2 cups cheddar cheese, shredded
- 1/2 cup salsa
- 1 lb ground sausage
- 1 1/2 cups coconut milk
- Pepper
- Salt

Directions:

1. Preheat the oven to 350° F.
2. Add sausage in a pan and cook until browned. Drain excess fat.
3. In a large bowl, whisk eggs and milk; add pepper and salt. Stir in cheese, cooked sausage, and salsa.
4. Pour omelet mixture into the baking dish and bake for 45 minutes.
5. Serve and enjoy.

Nutrition:

- Calories: 360
- Fat: 24 g
- Carbohydrates: 4 g
- Sugar: 3 g
- Protein: 28 g
- Cholesterol: 400 mg
- Sodium: 159 mg
- Potassium: 129 mg
- Phosphorous: 175 mg

Feta Mint Omelette

Preparation time: 10 minutes

Cooking time: 5 minutes

Servings: 1

Ingredients:

- 2 eggs
- 1/4 cup fresh mint, chopped
- 2 tbsp coconut milk
- 1/2 tsp olive oil
- 2 tbsp feta cheese, crumbled
- Pepper
- Salt

Directions:

1. In a bowl, whisk eggs with feta cheese, mint, milk, pepper and salt.

2. Heat olive oil in a pan over low heat.

3. Pour egg mixture in the pan and cook until eggs are set.

4. Flip omelet and cook for 2 minutes more.

5. Serve and enjoy.

Nutrition:

- Calories: 275
- Fat: 20 g
- Carbohydrates: 4 g
- Sugar: 2 g
- Protein: 20 g

- Cholesterol: 505 mg
- Sodium: 195 mg
- Potassium: 164 mg
- Phosphorous: 156 mg

Sausage Breakfast Casserole

Preparation time: 10 minutes

Cooking time: 50 minutes

Servings: 8

Ingredients:

- 12 eggs

- 1 lb. Italian ground sausage

- 2 1/2 tomatoes, sliced

- 3 tbsp coconut flour

- 1/4 cup coconut milk

- 2 small zucchinis, shredded

- Pepper

- Salt

Directions:

1. Preheat the oven to 350° F.

2. Spray casserole dish with cooking spray and set aside.

3. Cook sausage in a pan until brown.

4. Transfer sausage to a mixing bowl.

5. Add coconut flour, milk, eggs, zucchini, pepper and salt. Stir well.

6. Add eggs and whisk to combine.

7. Transfer the bowl mixture into the casserole dish and top with tomato slices.

8. Bake for 50 minutes.

9. Serve and enjoy.

Nutrition:

- Calories: 305
- Fat: 21.8 g
- Carbohydrates: 6.3 g
- Sugar: 3.3 g
- Protein: 19.6 g
- Cholesterol: 286 mg
- Sodium: 194 mg
- Potassium: 144 mg
- Phosphorous: 159 mg

Healthy Spinach Tomato Muffins

Preparation time: 10 minutes

Cooking time: 20 minutes

Servings: 12

Ingredients:

- 12 eggs
- 1/2 tsp Italian seasoning
- 1 cup tomatoes, chopped
- 4 tbsp water
- 1 cup fresh spinach, chopped
- Pepper
- Salt

Directions:

1. Preheat the oven to 350° F.
2. Spray a muffin tray with cooking spray and set aside.
3. In a mixing bowl, whisk eggs with water, Italian seasoning, pepper and salt.
4. Add spinach and tomatoes and stir well.
5. Pour egg mixture into the prepared muffin tray and bake for 20 minutes.
6. Serve and enjoy.

Nutrition:

- Calories: 67
- Fat: 4.5 g
- Carbohydrates: 1 g
- Sugar: 0.8 g
- Protein: 5.7 g
- Cholesterol: 164 mg
- Sodium: 114 mg
- Potassium: 193 mg
- Phosphorous: 140 mg

Pineapple Bread

Preparation time: 20 minutes

Cooking time: 1 hour

Servings: 10

Ingredients:

- 1/3 cup Swerve
- 1/3 cup butter, unsalted
- 2 eggs
- 2 cups flour
- 3 teaspoons baking powder
- 1 cup pineapple, undrained
- 6 cherries, chopped

Directions:

1. Whisk the Swerve with the butter in a mixer until fluffy.
2. Stir in the eggs; then, beat again.
3. Add the baking powder and flour; then, mix well until smooth.
4. Fold in the cherries and pineapple.
5. Spread this cherry-pineapple batter in a 9x5 inch baking pan.
6. Bake the pineapple batter for 1 hour at 350° F.
7. Slice the bread and serve.

Nutrition:

- Calories: 197
- Total Fat: 7.2g
- Saturated Fat: 1.3g
- Cholesterol: 33mg
- Sodium: 85mg
- Carbohydrates: 18.3g
- Dietary Fiber: 1.1g
- Sugar: 3 g
- Protein: 4g
- Calcium: 79mg
- Phosphorus: 144mg
- Potassium: 142mg

Apple Cinnamon Rings

Preparation time: 10 minutes

Cooking time: 20 minutes

Servings: 6

Ingredients:

- 4 large apples, cut in rings
- 1 cup flour
- 1/4 teaspoon baking powder
- 1 teaspoon stevia
- 1/4 teaspoon cinnamon
- 1 large egg, beaten
- 1 cup coconut milk
- Vegetable oil, for frying

Cinnamon Topping:

- 1/3 cup of brown Swerve
- 2 teaspoons cinnamon

Directions:

1. Begin by mixing the flour with the baking powder, cinnamon and stevia in a bowl.
2. Whisk the egg with the milk in a bowl.
3. Stir in the dry flour mixture and mix well until it makes a smooth batter.
4. Pour oil into a wok to deep fry the rings and heat it to 375 ° F.
5. First, dip the apple in the flour batter and deep fry until golden brown.
6. Transfer the apple rings to a tray lined with a paper towel.
7. Drizzle the cinnamon and Swerve topping over the slices.
8. Serve fresh in the morning.

Nutrition:

- Calories: 166
- Total Fat: 1.7g
- Saturated Fat: 0.5g
- Cholesterol: 33mg
- Sodium: 55mg
- Carbohydrates: 13.1g
- Dietary Fiber: 1.9g
- Sugar: 6.9g
- Protein: 4.7g
- Calcium: 65mg
- Phosphorus: 105mg
- Potassium: 197mg

Zucchini Bread

Preparation time: 20 minutes

Cooking time: 1 hour

Servings: 16

Ingredients:

- 3 eggs
- 1 1/2 cups Swerve
- 1 cup apple sauce
- 2 cups zucchini, shredded
- 1 teaspoon vanilla
- 2 cups flour
- 1/4 teaspoon baking powder
- 1 teaspoon baking soda
- 1 teaspoon cinnamon
- 1/2 teaspoon ginger
- 1 cup unsalted nuts, chopped

Directions:

1. Thoroughly whisk the eggs with the zucchini, apple sauce, and the rest of the ingredients in a bowl.
2. Once mixed evenly, spread the mixture in a loaf pan.
3. Bake it for 1 hour at 375° F in a preheated oven.
4. Slice and serve.

Nutrition:

- Calories: 200
- Total Fat: 5.4g
- Saturated Fat: 0.9g
- Cholesterol: 31mg
- Sodium: 94mg
- Carbohydrates: 26.9g
- Dietary Fiber: 1.6g
- Sugar: 16.3g
- Protein: 4.4g
- Calcium: 20mg
- Phosphorus: 100mg
- Potassium: 137 mg

Cauliflower Rice and Coconut

Preparation time: 20 minutes

Cooking time: 20 minutes

Servings: 4

Ingredients:

- 3 cups cauliflower, riced
- 2/3 cups full-fat coconut milk
- 1-2 teaspoons sriracha paste
- 1/4- 1/2 teaspoon onion powder
- Salt as needed
- Fresh basil for garnish

Directions:

1. Take a pan and place it over medium-low heat.

2. Add all of the ingredients and stir them until fully combined.

3. Cook for about 5–10 minutes, making sure that the lid is on.

4. Remove the lid and keep cooking until there's no excess liquid.

5. Once the rice is soft and creamy, enjoy it!

Nutrition:

- Calories: 95
- Fat: 7g
- Carbohydrates: 4g
- Protein: 1g
- Sodium: 39 mg
- Potassium: 169 mg
- Phosphorous: 78 mg

Soups and First Courses

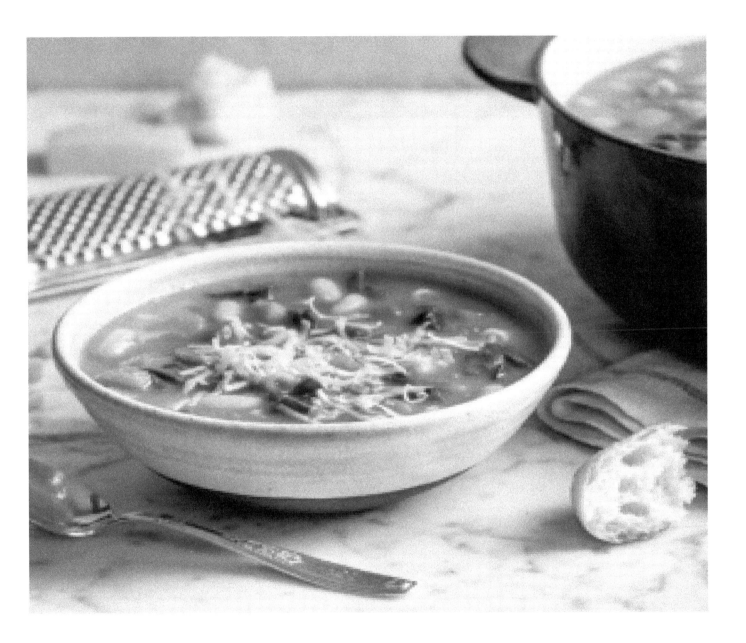

Chicken Wild Rice Soup

Preparation time: 10 minutes

Cooking time: 15 minutes

Servings: 6

Ingredients:

- 2/3 cup wild rice, uncooked
- 1 tbsp onion, chopped finely
- 1 cup carrots, chopped
- 8 oz chicken breast, cooked
- 2 tbsp butter
- 1/4 cup all-purpose white flour
- 5 cups low-sodium chicken broth
- 1 tbsp slivered almonds

Directions:

1. Start by adding rice and 2 cups broth along with 1/2 cup water to a cooking pot.

2. Cook until the rice is al dente and set it aside.

3. Add butter to a saucepan and melt it.

4. Stir in onion and sauté until soft, then add the flour and the remaining broth.

5. Stir and cook for 1 minute, then add the chicken, cooked rice and carrots.

6. Cook for 5 minutes on simmer.

7. Garnish with almonds.

8. Serve fresh.

Nutrition:

- Calories: 287
- Protein: 21 g
- Carbohydrates: 35 g
- Fat: 7 g
- Cholesterol: 42 mg
- Sodium: 182 mg
- Potassium: 101 mg
- Phosphorus 118 mg
- Calcium: 45 mg
- Fiber: 1.6 g

Chicken Noodle Soup

Preparation time: 10 minutes

Cooking time: 25 minutes

Servings: 2

Ingredients:

- 1 1/2 cups low-sodium vegetable broth
- 1 cup water
- 1/4 tsp poultry seasoning
- 1/4 tsp black pepper
- 1 cup chicken strips
- 1/4 cup carrot
- 2 oz egg noodles, uncooked

Directions:

1. Toss all the ingredients into a slow cooker

2. Cook soup on high heat for 25 minutes.

3. Serve warm.

Nutrition:

- Calories: 103
- Protein: 8 g
- Carbohydrates: 11 g
- Fat: 3 g
- Cholesterol: 4 mg
- Sodium: 176 mg
- Potassium: 164 mg
- Phosphorus: 128 mg
- Calcium: 46 mg
- Fiber: 4.0 g

Cucumber Soup

Preparation time: 10 minutes

Cooking time: 0 minutes

Servings: 4

Ingredients:

- 2 medium cucumbers, peeled and diced
- 1/3 cup sweet white onion, diced
- 1 green onion, diced
- 1/4 cup fresh mint
- 2 tbsp fresh dill
- 2 tbsp lemon juice
- 2/3 cup water
- 1/2 cup half and half cream
- 1/3 cup sour cream
- 1/2 tsp pepper
- Fresh dill sprigs for garnish

Directions:

1. Toss all the ingredients into a food processor.
2. Puree the mixture and refrigerate for 2 hours.
3. Garnish with dill sprigs.
4. Enjoy fresh.

Nutrition:

- Calories: 77
- Protein: 2 g
- Carbohydrates: 6 g
- Fat: 5 g
- Cholesterol: 12 mg
- Sodium: 128 mg
- Potassium: 158 mg
- Phosphorus: 102 mg
- Calcium: 60 mg
- Fiber: 1.0 g

Squash and Turmeric Soup

Preparation time: 10 minutes

Cooking time: 30 minutes

Servings: 4

Ingredients:

- 4 cups low-sodium vegetable broth
- 2 medium zucchini squash, peeled and diced
- 2 medium yellow crookneck squash, peeled and diced
- 1 small onion, diced
- 1/2 cup frozen green peas
- 2 tbsps olive oil
- 1/2 cup plain nonfat Greek yogurt
- 2 tsps turmeric

Directions:

1. Warm the broth in a saucepan on medium heat.

2. Toss in onion, squash, and zucchini.

3. Let it simmer for approximately 25 minutes, then add oil and green peas.

4. Cook for another 5 minutes, then allow it to cool.

5. Puree the soup using a handheld blender, then add Greek yogurt and turmeric.

6. Refrigerate it overnight and serve fresh.

Nutrition:

- Calories: 100
- Protein: 4 g
- Carbohydrates: 10 g
- Fat: 5 g
- Cholesterol: 1 mg
- Sodium: 168 mg
- Potassium: 104 mg
- Phosphorus: 138 mg
- Calcium: 60 mg
- Fiber: 2.8 g

Wild Rice Asparagus Soup

Preparation time: 10 minutes

Cooking time: 30 minutes

Servings: 4

Ingredients:

- 3/4 cup wild rice
- 2 cups asparagus, chopped
- 1 cup carrots, diced
- 1/2 cup onion, diced
- 3 cloves of garlic, minced
- 1/4 cup unsalted butter
- 1/2 tsp thyme
- 1/2 tsp fresh ground pepper
- 1/4 tsp nutmeg
- 1 bay leaf
- 1/2 cup all-purpose flour
- 4 cups low-sodium chicken broth
- 1/2 cup extra dry vermouth
- 2 cups cooked chicken
- 4 cups unsweetened almond milk, unenriched

Directions:

1. Cook the wild rice as per the cooking instructions on the box or bag and drain.

2. Melt the butter in a Dutch oven and sauté garlic and onion.

3. Once soft, add spices, herbs and carrots.

4. Cook on medium heat right until veggies are tender, then add flour and stir cook for 10 minutes on low heat.

5. Add 4 cups of broth and vermouth and blend using a handheld blender.

6. Dice the chicken pieces and add asparagus and chicken to the soup.

7. Stir in almond milk and cook for 20 minutes.

8. Add the wild rice and serve warm.

Nutrition:

- Calories: 295
- Protein: 21 g
- Carbohydrates: 28 g
- Fat: 11 g
- Cholesterol: 45 mg
- Sodium: 117 mg
- Potassium: 127 mg
- Phosphorus: 150 mg
- Calcium: 183 mg
- Fiber: 3.3 g

Nutmeg Chicken Soup

Preparation time: 10 minutes

Cooking time: 20 minutes

Servings: 4

Ingredients:

- 1 lb boneless, skinless chicken breasts, uncooked
- 1 1/2 cups onion, sliced
- 1 tbsp olive oil
- 1 cup fresh carrots, chopped
- 1 cup fresh green beans, chopped
- 3 tbsp all-purpose white flour
- 1 tsp dried oregano
- 2 tsp dried basil
- 1/4 tsp nutmeg
- 1 tsp thyme
- 32 oz reduced-sodium chicken broth
- 1/2 cup 1% low-fat milk
- 2 cups frozen green peas
- 1/4 tsp black pepper

Directions:

1. Add chicken to a skillet and sauté for 6 minutes, then remove it from the heat.

2. Warm-up olive oil in a pan and sauté onion for 5 minutes.

3. Stir in green beans, carrots, chicken, basil, oregano, flour, thyme and nutmeg.

4. Sauté for 3 minutes, then transfer the ingredients to a large pan.

5. Add milk and broth and cook until it boils.

6. Stir in green peas and cook for 5 minutes.

7. Adjust seasoning with pepper and serve warm.

Nutrition:

- Calories: 131
- Protein: 14 g
- Carbohydrates: 12 g
- Fat: 3 g
- Cholesterol: 32 mg
- Sodium: 194 mg
- Potassium: 167 mg
- Phosphorus: 135 mg
- Calcium: 67 mg
- Fiber: 2.8 g

Hungarian Cherry Soup

Preparation time: 10 minutes

Cooking time: 15 minutes

Servings: 4

Ingredients:

- 1 1/2 cup fresh cherries
- 3 cups water
- 1/3 cup sugar
- 1/16 tsp salt
- 1 tbsp all-purpose white flour
- 1/2 cup reduced-fat sour cream

Directions:

1. Warm the water in a saucepan and add cherries, salt and sugar.

2. Let it boil, then simmer for 10 minutes.

3. Remove 2 tbsp of the cooking liquid and keep it aside.

4. Separate 1/4 cup of liquid in a bowl and allow it to cool.

5. Add flour and sour cream to this liquid.

6. Mix well, then return the mixture to the saucepan.

7. Cook for 5 minutes on low heat.

8. Garnish the soup with the reserved 2 tbsp of liquid.

9. Serve and enjoy.

Nutrition:

- Calories: 144
- Protein: 2 g
- Carbohydrates: 25 g
- Fat: 4 g
- Cholesterol: 12 mg
- Sodium: 57 mg
- Potassium: 144 mg
- Phosphorus: 40 mg
- Calcium: 47 mg
- Fiber: 1.0 g

Italian Wedding Soup

Preparation time: 10 minutes

Cooking time: 10 minutes

Servings: 4

Ingredients:

- 1 lb lean ground beef
- 2 eggs
- 1/4 cup dried breadcrumbs
- 2 tbsp parmesan cheese, grated
- 1 tsp dried basil
- 3 tbsp onion, chopped
- 2 1/2 quarts low-sodium chicken broth
- 1 cup fresh spinach leaves
- 1 cup Acini di Pepe pasta, uncooked
- 3/4 cup carrots, chopped

Directions:

1. Start by tossing the eggs, beef, cheese, crumbs, onion and basil in a bowl.

2. Mix it well; then, make a half-inch thick log and slice it into 80 pieces.

3. Roll the meat slices into meatballs.

4. Warm the broth in a stockpot, then add pasta, spinach, carrots and meatballs.

5. Bring it to a boil, then simmer for 10 minutes on low heat.

6. Once it's done, serve warm.

Nutrition:

- Calories: 165
- Protein: 21 g
- Carbohydrates: 11 g
- Fat: 6 g
- Cholesterol: 73 mg
- Sodium: 191 mg
- Potassium: 181 mg
- Phosphorus: 146 mg
- Calcium: 42 mg
- Fiber: 1.0 g

Salmon Stuffed Pasta

Preparation time: 20 minutes

Cooking time: 35 minutes

Servings: 2

Ingredients:

- 24 jumbo pasta shells, boiled
- 1 cup coffee creamer

Filling:

- 2 eggs, beaten
- 2 cups creamed cottage cheese
- 1/4 cup chopped onion
- 1 red bell pepper, diced
- 2 teaspoons dried parsley
- 1/2 teaspoon lemon peel
- 1 can salmon, drained

Dill Sauce:

- 1 1/2 teaspoon butter
- 1 1/2 teaspoon flour
- 1/8 teaspoon pepper
- 1 tablespoon lemon juice
- 1 1/2 cup coffee creamer
- 2 teaspoons dried dill weed

Directions:

1. Beat the egg with the cream cheese and all the other filling ingredients in a bowl.
2. Divide the filling in the pasta shells and place the shells in a 9x13 baking dish.
3. Pour the coffee creamer around the stuffed shells; then cover with a foil.
4. Bake the shells for 30 minutes at 350° F.
5. Meanwhile, whisk all the ingredients for dill sauce in a saucepan.
6. Stir for 5 minutes until it thickens.
7. Pour this sauce over the baked pasta shells.
8. Serve warm.

Nutrition:

- Calories: 268
- Total Fat: 4.8g
- Sodium: 86mg
- Protein: 11.5g
- Calcium: 27mg
- Phosphorus: 192mg
- Potassium: 181mg

Old Fashioned Salmon Soup

Preparation time: 10 minutes

Cooking time: 20 minutes

Servings: 4

Ingredients:

- 2 tbsp unsalted butter
- 1 medium carrot, diced
- 1/2 cup celery, chopped
- 1/2 cup onion, sliced
- 1 lb sockeye salmon, cooked, diced
- 2 cups reduced-sodium chicken broth
- 2 cups 1% almond milk
- 1/8 tsp black pepper
- 1/4 cup cornstarch
- 1/4 cup water

Directions:

1. Melt butter in a saucepan and sauté all the vegetables in it until soft.
2. Stir in salmon chunks, milk, pepper, and broth.
3. Bring it to a boil, then simmer on low heat.
4. Mix cornstarch with water in a bowl and add this slurry to the soup.
5. Cook and stir continuously until it thickens.
6. Serve fresh and warm.

Nutrition:

- Calories: 155
- Protein: 14 g
- Carbohydrates: 9 g
- Fat: 7 g
- Cholesterol: 37 mg
- Sodium: 113 mg
- Potassium: 169 mg
- Phosphorus: 118 mg
- Calcium: 92 mg
- Fiber: 0.5 g

Oxtail Soup

Preparation time: 10 minutes

Cooking time: 20 minutes

Servings: 4

Ingredients:

- 1 medium bell pepper, diced
- 1 small jalapeno pepper, diced
- 1 large onion, sliced
- 3 celery stalks, chopped
- 1 tbsp olive oil
- 1 tbsp all-purpose white flour
- 2 bouillon cubes
- 2-lb package oxtail
- 1 tbsp vinegar
- 1/4 tsp black pepper
- 1/2 tsp herb seasoning blend
- 12 oz frozen gumbo vegetables

Directions:

1. Start by adding olive oil, flour, and the bouillon cubes to a saucepan.

2. Add water 3/4 of the way up the saucepan and let it boil.

3. Stir in peppers, vinegar, and oxtails.

4. Cover it and cook until the oxtails soften.

5. Add all vegetables including, celery and onion to the soup.

6. Cook until the veggies soften.

7. Serve fresh and warm.

Nutrition:

- Calories: 313
- Protein: 21 g
- Carbohydrates: 10 g
- Fat: 21 g
- Cholesterol: 66 mg

- Sodium: 125 mg
- Potassium: 196 mg
- Phosphorus: 149 mg
- Calcium: 61 mg
- Fiber: 2.2 g

Chicken and Corn Soup

Preparation time: 15 minutes

Cooking time: 60 minutes

Servings: 12

Ingredients:

- 6 ounces flat noodles, medium-sized, cooked
- 4-pound roasting chicken
- 10 ounces cooked corn

- 1/4 teaspoon ground black pepper
- 1 tablespoon parsley, chopped
- 14 cups water

Directions:

1. Take a large pot, place it over medium heat, pour in 8 cups water, add chicken, cook for 30 to 40 minutes until the chicken has cooked, and when done, separate chicken from broth and set aside until needed.

2. Meanwhile, cook the noodles until tender, omit the salt and when cooked, drain the noodles and set aside until required.

3. Remove fat from the chicken broth by skimming it, let the chicken cool slightly, and then cut it into bite-size pieces.

4. Take a large pot, place it over medium heat, pour in broth and remaining water, stir in chicken, add cooked noodles and corn, stir in black pepper and parsley and simmer for 15 to 20 minutes until hot.

5. When done, ladle soup into bowls and then serve.

Nutrition:

- Calories: 222
- Fat: 6 g
- Protein: 25 g
- Carbohydrates: 17 g
- Fiber: 1.4 g
- Cholesterol: 67 ml
- Sodium: 178 mg
- Potassium: 103 mg
- Phosphorous: 123 mg

Asparagus, Chicken and Wild Rice Soup

Preparation time: 10 minutes

Cooking time: 45 minutes

Servings: 8

Ingredients:

- 2 cups cooked chicken
- ¾ cup wild rice and white rice blend, cooked
- 1/2 cup all-purpose white flour
- 2 cups asparagus, diced
- 1 cup carrots, diced
- 1/2 cup white onion, diced
- 1 1/2 teaspoon minced garlic
- 1/2 teaspoon salt
- 1/2 teaspoon dried thyme
- 1/2 teaspoon ground black pepper
- 1/2 teaspoon ground nutmeg
- 1 bay leaf
- 1/4 cup unsalted butter
- 1/2 cup dry vermouth
- 4 cups chicken broth, low-sodium
- 4 cups almond milk, unenriched, unsweetened

Directions:

1. Take a Dutch oven, place it over medium heat, add butter and when it melts, add onion and garlic and cook for 5 minutes, or until tender.

2. Then add carrots, stir in all the spices and herbs and continue cooking for 5 minutes, or until carrots are tender.

3. Switch to low heat, stir in flour, continue cooking for 10 minutes, then pour in vermouth and chicken broth and whisk until combined.

4. Add chicken and asparagus, then gradually stir in milk and continue simmering for 20 minutes until cooked.

5. When done, fold rice into the soup and then serve.

Nutrition:

- Calories: 295
- Fat: 11 g
- Protein: 21 g
- Carbohydrates: 28 g
- Fiber: 3.3 g
- Cholesterol: 45 ml
- Potassium: 127 mg
- Sodium: 185 mg
- Phosphorous: 121 mg

Sausage & Egg Soup

Preparation time: 15 minutes

Cooking time: 30 minutes

Servings: 4

Ingredients:

- 1/2 lb. wheat
- Black pepper
- 1/2 teaspoon ground sage
- 1/2 teaspoon garlic powder
- 1/2 teaspoon dried basil
- 4 slices bread (one day old), cubed
- 2 tablespoons olive oil
- 1 tablespoon herb seasoning blend
- 2 cloves of garlic, minced
- 3 cups low-sodium chicken broth
- 1 cup water
- 4 tablespoons fresh parsley
- 4 eggs

Directions:

1. Preheat your oven to 375° F.

2. Mix the first five ingredients to make the sausage.

3. Toss bread cubes in oil and seasoning blend.

4. Bake in the oven for 8 minutes. Set aside.

5. Cook the sausage in a pan over medium heat.

6. Cook the garlic in the sausage drippings for 2 minutes.

7. Stir in the broth, water and parsley.

8. Bring to a boil and then simmer for 10 minutes.

9. Pour into serving bowls and top with baked bread, egg and sausage.

Nutrition:

- Calories: 335
- Protein: 26 g
- Carbohydrates: 15 g
- Fat: 19 g
- Cholesterol: 250 mg
- Sodium: 174 mg
- Potassium: 192 mg
- Phosphorus: 68 mg
- Calcium: 118 mg
- Fiber: 0.9 g

Spring Veggie Soup

Preparation time: 20 minutes

Cooking time: 45 minutes

Servings: 5

Ingredients:

- 2 tablespoons olive oil
- 1/2 cup onion, diced
- 1/2 cup mushrooms, sliced
- 1/8 cup celery, chopped
- 1 tomato, diced
- 1/2 cup carrots, diced
- 1 cup green beans, trimmed
- 1/2 cup frozen corn
- 1 teaspoon garlic powder
- 1 teaspoon dried oregano leaves
- 4 cups low-sodium vegetable broth

Directions:

1. In a pot, pour the olive oil and cook the onion and celery for 2 minutes.

2. Add the rest of the ingredients.

3. Bring to a boil.

4. Reduce heat and simmer for 45 minutes.

Nutrition:

- Calories: 114
- Protein: 2 g
- Carbohydrates: 13 g
- Fat: 6 g
- Cholesterol: 0 mg
- Sodium: 125 mg
- Potassium: 199 mg
- Phosphorus: 108 mg
- Calcium: 48 mg
- Fiber: 3.4 g

Delicious Vegetarian Lasagna

Preparation time: 10 minutes

Cooking time: 1 hour

Servings: 4

Ingredients:

- 1 teaspoon basil
- 1 tablespoon olive oil
- 1/2 sliced red pepper
- 3 lasagna sheets
- 1/2 diced red onion
- 1/4 teaspoon black pepper

- 1 cup rice milk
- 1 clove of garlic, minced
- 1 cup sliced eggplant
- 1/2 sliced zucchini
- 1/2 pack soft tofu
- 1 teaspoon oregano

Directions:

1. Preheat oven to 325°F/Gas Mark 3.

2. Slice zucchini, eggplant, and pepper into vertical strips.

3. Add the rice milk and tofu to a food processor and blitz until smooth. Set aside.

4. Heat the oil in a skillet over medium heat and add the onions and garlic for 3-4 minutes or until soft.

5. Sprinkle in the herbs and pepper and allow to stir through for 5-6 minutes until hot.

6. Into a lasagna or suitable oven dish, layer 1 lasagna sheet, then 1/3 the eggplant, followed by 1/3 zucchini, then 1/3 pepper before pouring over 1/3 of white tofu sauce.

7. Repeat for the next 2 layers, finishing with the white sauce.

8. Add to the oven for 40-50 minutes, or until veg is soft and can easily be sliced into servings.

Nutrition:

- Calories: 235
- Protein: 5 g
- Carbs: 10g
- Fat: 9 g

- Sodium: 35mg
- Potassium: 129mg
- Phosphorus: 66mg

Pasta Fagioli

Preparation time: 25 minutes

Cooking time: 25 minutes

Servings: 6

Ingredients:

- 1 (15-ounce) can low-sodium great northern beans, drained and rinsed, divided
- 2 cups frozen peppers and onions, thawed, divided
- 5 cups low-sodium vegetable broth
- 1/8 teaspoon salt
- 1/8 teaspoon freshly ground black pepper
- 1 cup whole-grain orecchiette pasta
- 2 tablespoons extra-virgin olive oil
- 1/3 cup grated Parmesan cheese

Directions:

1. In a large saucepan, place the beans and cover them with water. Bring to a boil over high heat and boil for 10 minutes. Drain the beans.

2. In a food processor or blender, combine 1/3 cup of beans and 1/3 cup of thawed peppers and onions. Process until smooth.

3. In the same saucepan, combine the pureed mixture, the remaining 1 2/3 cups of peppers and onions, the remaining beans, the broth, and the salt and pepper, and bring to a simmer.

4. Add the pasta to the saucepan. Make sure to stir it and bring it to boil, reduce the heat to low, and simmer for 8 to 10 minutes, or until the pasta is tender.

5. Serve drizzled with olive oil and topped with Parmesan cheese.

Nutrition:

- Calories: 245
- Total fat: 7g
- Saturated fat: 2g
- Sodium: 169mg
- Phosphorus: 144mg
- Potassium: 192mg
- Carbohydrates: 36g
- Fiber: 7g
- Protein: 12g
- Sugar: 4g

Cod & Green Bean Risotto

Preparation time: 4 minutes

Cooking time: 40 minutes

Servings: 2

Ingredients:

- 1/2 cup arugula
- 1 finely diced white onion
- 4 oz. cod fillet
- 1 cup white rice
- 2 lemon wedges
- 1 cup boiling water
- 1/4 tsp. black pepper
- 1 cup low sodium chicken broth
- 1 tbsp. extra virgin olive oil
- 1/2 cup green beans

Directions:

1. Heat the oil in a large pan on medium heat.
2. Sauté the chopped onion for 5 minutes until soft before adding in the rice and stirring for 1-2 minutes.
3. Combine the broth with boiling water.
4. Add half of the liquid to the pan and stir slowly.
5. Slowly add the rest of the liquid whilst continuously stirring for up to 20-30 minutes.
6. Stir in the green beans to the risotto.
7. Place the fish on top of the rice, cover and steam for 10 minutes.
8. Ensure the water does not dry out and keep topping up until the rice is cooked thoroughly.
9. Use your fork to break up the fish fillets and stir into the rice.
10. Sprinkle with freshly ground pepper to serve and a squeeze of fresh lemon.
11. Garnish with the lemon wedges and serve with the arugula.

Nutrition:

- Calories: 221
- Protein: 12 g
- Carbs: 29 g
- Fat: 8 g
- Sodium: 198 mg
- Potassium: 147 mg
- Phosphorus: 141 mg

Fish and Seafood

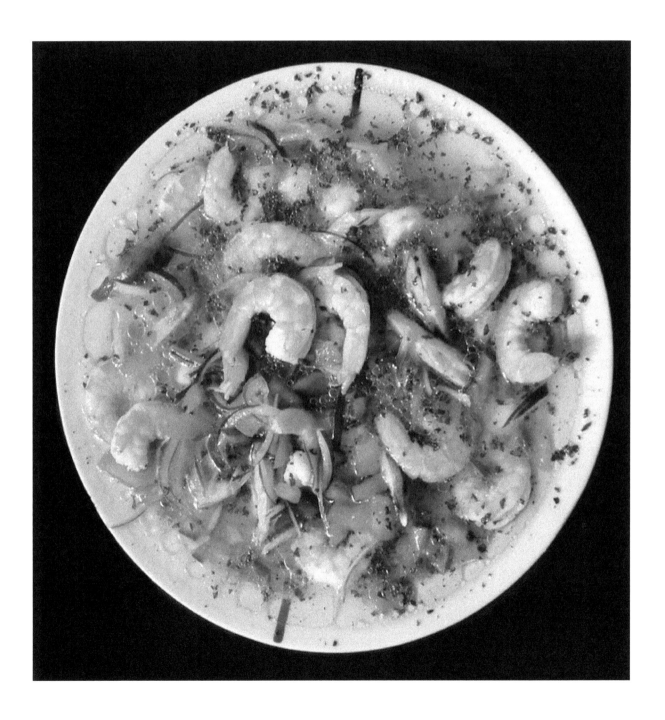

Salmon & Pesto Salad

Preparation time: 5 minutes

Cooking time: 15 minutes

Servings: 2

Ingredients:

For the pesto:

- 1 clove of garlic, minced
- 1/2 cup fresh arugula
- 1/4 cup extra virgin olive oil
- 1/2 cup fresh basil
- 1 tsp. black pepper

For the salmon:

- 4 oz. skinless salmon fillet
- 1 tbsp. coconut oil

For the salad:

- 1/2 juiced lemon
- 2 sliced radishes
- 1/2 cup iceberg lettuce
- 1 tsp. black pepper

Directions:

1. Prepare the pesto by blending all the ingredients for the pesto in a food processor or by grinding with a pestle and mortar. Set aside.

2. Add a skillet to the stove on medium-high heat and melt the coconut oil.

3. Add the salmon to the pan.

4. Cook for 7-8 minutes and turn over.

5. Cook for a further 3-4 minutes or until cooked through.

6. Remove fillets from the skillet and allow to rest.

7. Mix the lettuce and the radishes and squeeze over the juice of 1/2 lemon.

8. Flake the salmon with a fork and mix through the salad.

9. Toss to coat and sprinkle with a little black pepper to serve.

Nutrition:

- Calories: 221
- Protein: 13 g
- Carbs: 1 g
- Fat: 34 g
- Sodium: 80 mg
- Potassium: 119 mg
- Phosphorus: 148 mg

Baked Fennel & Garlic Sea Bass

Preparation time: 5 minutes

Cooking time: 15 minutes

Servings: 2

Ingredients:

- 1 lemon
- 1/2 sliced fennel bulb
- 6 oz. sea bass fillets
- 1 tsp. black pepper
- 2 cloves of garlic

Directions:

1. Preheat the oven to 375°F/Gas Mark 5.
2. Sprinkle black pepper over the Sea Bass.
3. Slice the fennel bulb and cloves of garlic.
4. Add 1 salmon fillet and half the fennel and garlic to one sheet of baking paper or tin foil.
5. Squeeze in 1/2 lemon juices.
6. Repeat for the other fillet.
7. Fold and add to the oven for 12-15 minutes or until fish is thoroughly cooked through.
8. Meanwhile, add boiling water to your couscous, cover and allow to steam.
9. Serve with your choice of rice or salad.

Nutrition:

- Calories: 221
- Protein: 14 g
- Carbs: 3 g
- Fat: 2 g
- Sodium: 119 mg
- Potassium: 198 mg
- Phosphorus: 149 mg

Lemon, Garlic & Cilantro Tuna and Rice

Preparation time: 5 minutes

Cooking time: 0 minutes

Servings: 2

Ingredients:

- 1/2 cup arugula
- 1 tbsp. extra virgin olive oil
- 1 cup cooked rice
- 1 tsp. black pepper
- 1/4 finely diced red onion
- 3 oz. canned tuna
- 2 tbsps. Chopped fresh cilantro

Directions:

1. Mix the olive oil, pepper, cilantro and red onion in a bowl.
2. Stir in the tuna, cover and leave in the fridge for as long as possible (if you can) or serve immediately.
3. When ready to eat, serve up with the cooked rice and arugula!

Nutrition:

- Calories: 221
- Protein: 11 g
- Carbs: 26 g
- Fat: 7 g
- Sodium: 143 mg
- Potassium: 197 mg
- Phosphorus: 132 mg

Sardine Fish Cakes

Preparation time: 10 minutes

Cooking time: 10 minutes

Servings: 4

Ingredients:

- 11 oz sardines, canned, drained
- 1/3 cup shallot, chopped
- 1 teaspoon chili flakes
- 1/2 teaspoon salt
- 2 tablespoons wheat flour, whole grain
- 1 egg, beaten
- 1 tablespoon chives, chopped
- 1 teaspoon olive oil
- 1 teaspoon butter

Directions:

1. Put the butter in the skillet and melt it.
2. Add shallot and cook it until translucent.
3. After this, transfer the shallot to the mixing bowl.
4. Add sardines, chili flakes, salt, flour, egg, chives and mix up until smooth with the help of the fork.
5. Make the medium size cakes and place them in the skillet.
6. Add olive oil.
7. Roast the fish cakes for 3 minutes from each side over medium heat.
8. Dry the cooked fish cakes with paper towel if needed and transfer them to the serving plates.

Nutrition:

- Calories: 221
- Fat: 12.2
- Fiber: 0.1
- Carbs: 5.4
- Protein: 21.3
- Sodium: 182 mg
- Potassium: 188 mg
- Phosphorous: 131 mg

Cajun Catfish

Preparation time: 10 minutes

Cooking time: 10 minutes

Servings:4

Ingredients:

- 16 oz catfish steaks (4 oz each fish steak)
- 1 tablespoon Cajun spices
- 1 egg, beaten
- 1 tablespoon sunflower oil

Directions:

1. Pour sunflower oil in the skillet and preheat it until shimmering.

2. Meanwhile, dip every catfish steak in the beaten egg and coat in Cajun spices.

3. Place the fish steaks in the hot oil and roast them for 4 minutes from each side.

4. The cooked catfish steaks should have a light brown crust.

Nutrition:

- Calories: 263
- Fat: 16.7
- Fiber: 0
- Carbs: 0.1
- Protein: 26.3
- Sodium: 100 mg
- Potassium: 180 mg
- Phosphorous: 141 mg

Salmon Fillet

Preparation time: 5 minutes

Cooking time: 25 minutes

Servings: 1

Ingredients:

- 4 oz salmon fillet
- 1/2 teaspoon salt
- 1 teaspoon sesame oil
- 1/2 teaspoon sage

Directions:

1. Rub the fillet with salt and sage.

2. Place the fish in the tray and sprinkle it with sesame oil.

3. Cook the fish for 25 minutes at 365°F.

4. Flip the fish carefully onto another side after 12 minutes of cooking.

Nutrition:

- Calories: 191
- Fat: 11.6
- Fiber: 0.1
- Carbs: 0.2

- Protein: 22
- Sodium: 154 mg
- Potassium: 178 mg
- Phosphorous: 154 mg

Spanish Cod in Sauce

Preparation time: 10 minutes

Cooking time: 5.5 hours

Servings: 2

Ingredients:

- 1 teaspoon tomato paste

- 1 teaspoon garlic, diced

- 1 white onion, sliced

- 1 jalapeno pepper, chopped

- 1/3 cup chicken stock

- 7 oz Spanish cod fillet

- 1 teaspoon paprika

- 1 teaspoon salt

Directions:

1. Pour chicken stock in the saucepan. Add tomato paste and mix up the liquid until homogenous.

2. Add garlic, onion, jalapeno pepper, paprika and salt.

3. Bring the liquid to boil and then simmer it.

4. Chop the cod fillet and add it to the tomato liquid. Close the lid and simmer the fish for 10 minutes over low heat.

5. Serve the fish in the bowls with tomato sauce.

Nutrition:

- Calories: 113
- Fat: 1.2
- Fiber: 1.9
- Carbs: 7.2

- Protein: 18.9
- Sodium: 169 mg
- Potassium: 103 mg
- Phosphorous: 65 mg

Fish Shakshuka

Preparation time: 5 minutes

Cooking time: 15 minutes

Servings: 5

Ingredients:

- 5 eggs
- 1 cup tomatoes, chopped
- 3 bell peppers, chopped
- 1 tablespoon butter
- 1 teaspoon tomato paste
- 1 teaspoon chili pepper
- 1 teaspoon salt
- 1 tablespoon fresh dill
- 5 oz cod fillet, chopped
- 1 tablespoon scallions, chopped

Directions:

1. Melt butter in the skillet and add chili pepper, bell peppers and tomatoes.
2. Sprinkle the vegetables with scallions, dill, salt, and chili pepper. Simmer them for 5 minutes.
3. After this, add chopped cod fillet and mix up well.
4. Close the lid and simmer the ingredients for 5 minutes over medium heat.
5. Then crack the eggs over the fish and close the lid.
6. Cook shakshuka with the closed lid for 5 minutes.

Nutrition:

- Calories: 143
- Fat: 7.3
- Fiber: 1.6
- Carbs: 7.9
- Protein: 12.8
- Sodium: 106 mg
- Potassium: 177 mg
- Phosphorous: 146 mg

Salmon Baked in Foil With Fresh Thyme

Preparation time: 10 minutes

Cooking time: 30 minutes

Servings:4

Ingredients:

- 4 fresh thyme sprigs
- 4 cloves of garlic, peeled, roughly chopped
- 16 oz salmon fillets (4 oz each fillet)
- 1/2 teaspoon salt
- 1/2 teaspoon ground black pepper
- 4 tablespoons cream
- 4 teaspoons butter
- 1/4 teaspoon cumin seeds

Directions:

1. Line the baking tray with foil.

2. Sprinkle the fish fillets with salt, ground black pepper, cumin seeds and arrange them in the tray with oil.

3. Add thyme sprig on the top of every fillet.

4. Then add cream, butter and garlic.

5. Bake the fish for 30 minutes at 345F.

Nutrition:

- Calories: 198
- Fat: 11.6
- Fiber: 0.2
- Carbs: 1.8
- Protein: 22.4
- Sodium: 119 mg
- Potassim: 126 mg
- Phosphorous: 135 mg

Poached Halibut in Orange Sauce

Preparation time: 10 minutes

Cooking time: 10 minutes

Servings: 4

Ingredients:

- 1-pound halibut
- 1/3 cup butter
- 1 rosemary sprig
- 1/2 teaspoon ground black pepper
- 1 teaspoon salt
- 1 teaspoon honey
- 1/4 cup orange juice
- 1 teaspoon cornstarch

Directions:

1. Put butter in the saucepan and melt it.
2. Add rosemary sprig.
3. Sprinkle the halibut with salt and ground black pepper.
4. Put the fish in the boiling butter and poach it for 4 minutes.
5. Meanwhile, pour orange juice in the skillet. Add honey and bring the liquid to boil.
6. Add cornstarch and whisk until the liquid starts to be thick.
7. Then remove it from the heat.
8. Transfer the poached halibut to the plate and cut it on 4.
9. Place every fish serving on the serving plate and top with orange sauce.

Nutrition:

- Calories: 349
- Fat: 29.3
- Fiber: 0.1
- Carbs: 3.2
- Protein: 17.8
- Sodium: 193 mg
- Potassium: 156 mg
- Phosphorous 144 mg

Fish en Papillote

Preparation time: 15 minutes

Cooking time: 20 minutes

Servings: 3

Ingredients:

- 10 oz snapper fillet
- 1 tablespoon fresh dill, chopped
- 1 white onion, peeled, sliced
- 1/2 teaspoon tarragon
- 1 tablespoon olive oil
- 1 teaspoon salt
- 1/2 teaspoon hot pepper
- 2 tablespoons sour cream

Directions:

1. Make the medium size packets from parchment and arrange them in the baking tray.
2. Cut the snapper fillet on 3 and sprinkle them with salt, tarragon, and hot pepper.
3. Put the fish fillets in the parchment packets.
4. Then top the fish with olive oil, sour cream sliced onion and fresh dill.
5. Bake the fish for 20 minutes at 355°F.

Nutrition:

- Calories: 204
- Fat: 8.2
- Fiber: 1
- Carbs: 4.6
- Protein: 27.2
- Sodium: 143 mg
- Potassium: 166 mg
- Phosphorous: 103 mg

Tuna Casserole

Preparation time: 15 minutes

Cooking time: 35 minutes

Servings:4

Ingredients:

- 1/2 cup Cheddar cheese, shredded
- 2 tomatoes, chopped
- 7 oz tuna filet, chopped
- 1 teaspoon ground coriander
- 1/2 teaspoon salt
- 1 teaspoon olive oil
- 1/2 teaspoon dried oregano

Directions:

1. Brush the casserole mold with olive oil.
2. Mix up together chopped tuna fillet with dried oregano, salt and ground coriander.
3. Place the fish in the mold and flatten well to get the layer.
4. Then add chopped tomatoes and shredded cheese.
5. Cover the casserole with foil and secure the edges.
6. Bake the meal for 35 minutes at 355°F.

Nutrition:

- Calories: 260
- Fat: 21.5
- Fiber: 0.8
- Carbs: 2.7
- Protein: 14.6
- Sodium: 116 mg
- Potassium: 137 mg
- Phosphorous: 84 mg

Oregano Salmon With Crunchy Crust

Preparation time: 10 minutes

Cooking time: 2 hours

Servings: 2

Ingredients:

- 8 oz salmon fillet
- 2 tablespoons panko breadcrumbs
- 1 oz Parmesan, grated
- 1 teaspoon dried oregano
- 1 teaspoon sunflower oil

Directions:

1. In the mixing bowl, combine panko breadcrumbs, Parmesan and dried oregano.
2. Sprinkle the salmon with oil and coat in the breadcrumb's mixture.
3. After this, line the baking tray with baking paper.
4. Place the salmon in the tray and transfer into the preheated oven at 385°F.
5. Bake the salmon for 25 minutes.

Nutrition:

- Calories: 245
- Fat: 12.8
- Fiber: 0.6
- Carbs: 5.9
- Protein: 27.5
- Sodium: 154 mg
- Potassium: 165 mg
- Phosphorous: 144 mg

Fish Chili With Lentils

Preparation time: 10 minutes

Cooking time: 30 minutes

Servings:4

Ingredients:

- 1 red pepper, chopped
- 1 yellow onion, diced
- 1 teaspoon ground black pepper
- 1 teaspoon butter
- 1 jalapeno pepper, chopped
- 1/2 cup lentils
- 3 cups chicken stock
- 1 teaspoon salt
- 1 tablespoon tomato paste
- 1 teaspoon chili pepper
- 8 oz cod, chopped

Directions:

1. Place butter, red pepper, onion, and ground black pepper in the saucepan.
2. Roast the vegetables for 5 minutes over medium heat.
3. Then add chopped jalapeno pepper, lentils and chili pepper.
4. Mix up the mixture well and add chicken stock and tomato paste.
5. Stir until homogenous. Add cod.
6. Close the lid and cook chili for 20 minutes over medium heat.

Nutrition:

- Calories: 187
- Fat: 2.3
- Fiber: 8.8
- Carbs: 21.3
- Protein: 20.6
- Sodium: 124 mg
- Potassium: 116 mg
- Phosphorous: 144 mg

Chili Mussels

Preparation time: 7 minutes

Cooking time: 10 minutes

Servings: 4

Ingredients:

- 1-pound mussels
- 1 chili pepper, chopped
- 1 cup chicken stock
- 1/2 cup almond milk
- 1 teaspoon olive oil
- 1 teaspoon minced garlic
- 1 teaspoon ground coriander
- 1/2 teaspoon salt
- 1 cup fresh parsley, chopped
- 4 tablespoons lemon juice

Directions:

1. Pour milk in the saucepan.
2. Add chili pepper, chicken stock, olive oil, minced garlic, ground coriander, salt and lemon juice.
3. Bring the liquid to boil and add mussels.
4. Boil the mussel for 4 minutes or until open the shells.
5. Then add chopped parsley and mix up the meal well.
6. Remove it from the heat.

Nutrition:

- Calories: 136
- Fat: 4.
- Fiber: 0.6
- Carbs: 7.5
- Protein: 15.3
- Sodium: 132 mg
- Potassium: 189 mg
- Phosphorous: 142 mg

Fried Scallops in Heavy Cream

Preparation time: 10 minutes

Cooking time: 7 minutes

Servings: 4

Ingredients:

- 1/2 cup heavy cream
- 1 teaspoon fresh rosemary
- 1/2 teaspoon dried cumin
- 1/2 teaspoon garlic, diced
- 8 oz bay scallops
- 1 teaspoon olive oil
- 1/2 teaspoon salt
- 1/4 teaspoon chili flakes

Directions:

1. Preheat olive oil in the skillet until hot.
2. Then sprinkle scallops with salt, chili flakes and dried cumin and place in the hot oil.
3. Add fresh rosemary and diced garlic.
4. Roast the scallops for 2 minutes from each side.
5. After this, add heavy cream and bring the mixture to boil. Boil it for 1 minute.

Nutrition:

- Calories: 114
- Fat: 7.3
- Fiber: 0.2
- Carbs: 2
- Protein: 9.9
- Sodium: 180 mg
- Potassium: 199 mg
- Phosphorous: 143 mg

Lettuce Seafood Wraps

Preparation time: 10 minutes

Cooking time: 0 minutes

Servings: 6

Ingredients:

- 6 lettuce leaves
- 8 oz salmon, canned
- 4 oz crab meat, canned
- 1 cucumber
- 2 tablespoons Plain yogurt
- 1/2 teaspoon minced garlic
- 1 tablespoon fresh dill, chopped
- 1/4 teaspoon tarragon

Directions:

1. Mash the salmon and crab meat with a fork.
2. Then add Plain yogurt, minced garlic, fresh dill and tarragon.
3. Grate the cucumber and add it to the seafood mixture. Mix up well.
4. Fill the lettuce leaves with a cooked mixture.

Nutrition:

- Calories: 80
- Fat: 2.8
- Fiber: 0.4
- Carbs: 3.1
- Protein: 10.5
- Sodium: 173 mg
- Potassium: 142 mg
- Phosphorous: 131 mg

Mango Tilapia Fillets

Preparation time: 10 minutes

Cooking time: 15 minutes

Servings: 4

Ingredients:

- 1/4 cup coconut flakes
- 5 oz mango, peeled
- 1/3 cup shallot, chopped
- 1 teaspoon ground turmeric
- 1 cup water
- 1 bay leaf
- 12 oz tilapia fillets
- 1 chili pepper, chopped
- 1 tablespoon coconut oil
- 1/2 teaspoon salt
- 1 teaspoon paprika

Directions:

1. Blend together coconut flakes, mango, shallot, ground turmeric and water.
2. After this, melt coconut oil in the saucepan.
3. Sprinkle the tilapia fillets with salt and paprika.
4. Then place them in the hot coconut oil and roast for 1 minute from each side.
5. Add chili pepper, bay leaf, and blended mango mixture.
6. Close the lid and cook fish for 10 minutes over medium heat.

Nutrition:

- Calories: 153
- Fat: 6.1
- Fiber: 1.5
- Carbs: 9.3
- Protein: 16.8
- Sodium: 154 mg
- Potassium: 122 mg
- Phosphorous: 148 mg

Omega-3 Rich Salmon

Preparation time: 10 minutes

Cooking time: 20-25 minutes

Servings: 2

Ingredients:

- 2 (4-ounce) skinless, boneless salmon fillets
- 2 tbsp. fresh lemon juice
- 1 tbsp. olive oil
- 1/4 tsp. crushed dried oregano
- Pinch salt
- Freshly ground black pepper, to taste

Directions:

1. Preheat the oven to 425°F. Line a baking sheet with parchment paper.

2. Place the salmon fillets onto the prepared baking sheet.

3. Drizzle with lemon juice and oil evenly and sprinkle with oregano, salt and black pepper.

4. Bake for about 20–25 minutes.

5. Serve hot.

Nutrition:

- Calories: 265
- Fat: 19.2g
- Carbs: 0.5g
- Protein: 22.3g
- Fiber: 0g
- Potassium: 23mg
- Sodium: 146mg
- Phosphorous: 1 mg

Wholesome Salmon Meal

Preparation time: 10 minutes

Cooking time: 20–25 minutes

Servings: 6

Ingredients:

- 4 (6-ounce) (1-inch thick) skinless salmon fillets
- Freshly ground black pepper, to taste
- 2 cups finely chopped zucchini, chopped finely
- 1 cup halved cherry tomatoes
- 1 tbsp. olive oil
- 1 tbsp. fresh lemon juice

Directions:

1. Preheat the oven to 425°F. Grease an 11x7-inch baking sheet.
2. Place the salmon fillets in the prepared baking sheet in a single layer and sprinkle with black pepper generously.
3. In a bowl, mix the remaining ingredients.
4. Place the mixture over salmon fillets evenly.
5. Bake for about 22 minutes.
6. Remove from the oven and keep aside to cool slightly.
7. Cut the salmon into small chunks and mix with the veggie mixture.
8. Serve warm.

Nutrition:

- Calories: 233
- Fat: 14.5g
- Carbs: 2.5g
- Protein: 22.9g
- Fiber: 0.8g
- Potassium: 173mg
- Sodium: 71mg
- Phosphorous: 15 mg

Succulent Tilapia

Preparation time: 10 minutes

Cooking time: 12–15 minutes

Servings: 4

Ingredients:

- 2 tbsp. unsalted margarine
- 4 cloves of garlic, minced
- 1 tsp. chopped fresh parsley
- Freshly ground black pepper, to taste
- Pinch Mrs. Dash salt-free herb seasoning
- 4 (4-ounce) tilapia fillets

Directions:

1. Preheat the oven to 350°F. Line a shallow baking sheet with a piece of foil.
2. In a large nonstick skillet, add margarine, garlic, parsley, black pepper and seasoning on low heat.
3. Cook till melted completely, stirring continuously.
4. Remove from heat.
5. At the bottom of a prepared baking sheet, spread a little of the garlic sauce evenly.
6. Arrange the tilapia fillets over the garlic sauce.
7. Coat the top of each tilapia fillet with the garlic sauce evenly.
8. Bake for about 12–15 minutes.

Nutrition:

- Calories: 149
- Fat: 6.7g
- Carbs: 1.1g
- Protein: 21.4g
- Fiber: 0g
- Potassium: 17mg
- Sodium: 107mg
- Phosphorous: 102 mg

Festive Tilapia

Preparation time: 10 minutes

Cooking time: 3 minutes

Servings: 8

Ingredients:

- 1/3 cup shredded low-fat Parmesan cheese
- 2 tbsp. low-sodium mayonnaise
- 1/4 cup softened unsalted butter
- 2 tbsp. fresh lemon juice
- 2 pounds tilapia fillets
- 1/4 tsp. crushed dried thyme
- Freshly ground black pepper, to taste

Directions:

1. Preheat the broiler. Grease the broiler pan.
2. In a large bowl, mix all ingredients except tilapia fillets. Keep aside.
3. Place the fillets onto the prepared broiler pan in a single layer.
4. Broil the fillets for about 2–3 minutes.
5. Remove from the oven and top the fillets with cheese mixture evenly.
6. Broil for about 2 minutes more.

Nutrition:

- Calories: 176
- Fat: 9.1g
- Carbs: 1.2g
- Protein: 22.9g
- Fiber: 0g
- Potassium: 7mg
- Sodium: 108mg
- Phosphorous: 120 mg

Herbed Vegetable Trout

Preparation time: 15 minutes

Cooking time: 15 minutes

Servings: 4

Ingredients:

- 14 oz. trout fillets
- 1/2 teaspoon herb seasoning blend
- 1 lemon, sliced
- 2 green onions, sliced
- 1 stalk celery, chopped
- 1 medium carrot, julienne

Directions:

1. Prepare and preheat a charcoal grill over moderate heat.
2. Place the trout fillets over a large piece of foil and drizzle herb seasoning on top.
3. Spread the lemon slices, carrots, celery, and green onions over the fish.
4. Cover the fish with foil and pack it.
5. Place the packed fish in the grill and cook for 15 minutes.
6. Once done, remove the foil from the fish.
7. Serve.

Nutrition:

- Calories: 202
- Total Fat: 8.5g
- Sodium: 82mg
- Calcium: 70mg
- Phosphorus: 150mg
- Potassium: 160mg

Citrus Glazed Salmon

Preparation time: 20 minutes

Cooking time: 17 minutes

Servings: 4

Ingredients:

- 2 cloves of garlic, crushed
- 1 1/2 tablespoons lemon juice
- 2 tablespoons olive oil
- 1 tablespoon butter
- 1 tablespoon Dijon mustard
- 2 dashes cayenne pepper
- 1 teaspoon dried basil leaves
- 1 teaspoon dried dill
- 24 oz. salmon filet

Directions:

1. Place a 1-quart saucepan over moderate heat and add the oil, butter, garlic, lemon juice, mustard, cayenne pepper, dill and basil to the pan.
2. Stir this mixture for 5 minutes after it has boiled.
3. Prepare and preheat a charcoal grill over moderate heat.
4. Place the fish on a foil sheet and fold the edges to make a foil tray.
5. Pour the prepared sauce over the fish.
6. Place the fish in the foil in the preheated grill and cook for 12 minutes.
7. Slice and serve.

Nutrition:

- Calories: 401
- Total Fat: 20.5g
- Cholesterol: 144mg
- Sodium: 155mg
- Carbohydrates: 0.5g
- Calcium: 549mg
- Phosphorus: 126mg
- Potassium: 146mg

Broiled Salmon Fillets

Preparation time: 10 minutes

Cooking time: 13 minutes

Servings: 4

Ingredients:

- 1 tablespoon ginger root, grated
- 1 clove of garlic, minced
- 1/4 cup maple syrup
- 1 tablespoon hot pepper sauce
- 4 salmon fillets, skinless

Directions:

1. Grease a pan with cooking spray and place it over moderate heat.
2. Add the ginger and garlic and sauté for 3 minutes, then transfer to a bowl.
3. Add the hot pepper sauce and maple syrup to the ginger-garlic.
4. Mix well and keep this mixture aside.
5. Place the salmon fillet in a suitable baking tray, greased with cooking oil.
6. Brush the maple sauce over the fillets liberally
7. Broil them for 10 minutes in the oven at broiler settings.
8. Serve warm.

Nutrition:

- Calories: 289
- Total Fat: 11.1g
- Sodium: 80mg
- Carbohydrates: 13.6g
- Calcium: 78mg
- Phosphorus: 2mg
- Potassium: 56mg

Broiled Shrimp

Preparation time: 10 minutes

Cooking time: 5 minutes

Servings: 8

Ingredients:

- 1 lb. shrimp in shell
- 1/2 cup unsalted butter, melted
- 2 teaspoons lemon juice
- 2 tablespoons chopped onion
- 1 clove of garlic, minced
- 1/8 teaspoon pepper

Directions:

1. Toss the shrimp with the butter, lemon juice, onion, garlic, and pepper in a bowl.
2. Spread the seasoned shrimp in a baking tray.
3. Broil for 5 minutes in an oven on a broiler setting.
4. Serve warm.

Nutrition:

- Calories: 164
- Total Fat: 12.8g
- Sodium: 142mg
- Carbohydrates: 0.6g
- Calcium: 45mg
- Phosphorus: 117mg
- Potassium: 64mg

Grilled Lemony Cod

Preparation time: 10 minutes

Cooking time: 10 minutes

Servings: 4

Ingredients:

- 1 lb. cod fillets
- 1 teaspoon salt-free lemon pepper seasoning
- 1/4 cup lemon juice

Directions:

1. Rub the cod fillets with lemon pepper seasoning and lemon juice.
2. Grease a baking tray with cooking spray and place the salmon in the baking tray.
3. Bake the fish for 10 minutes at 350 ° F in a preheated oven.
4. Serve warm.

Nutrition:

- Calories: 155
- Total Fat: 7.1g
- Cholesterol: 50mg
- Sodium: 53mg

- Protein: 22.2g
- Calcium: 43mg
- Phosphorus: 120mg
- Potassium: 182mg

Spiced Honey Salmon

Preparation time: 15 minutes

Cooking time: 16 minutes

Servings: 4

Ingredients:

- 3 tablespoons honey

- 3/4 teaspoon lemon peel

- 1/2 teaspoon black pepper

- 1/2 teaspoon garlic powder

- 1 teaspoon water

- 16 oz. salmon fillets

- 2 tablespoons olive oil

- Dill, chopped, to serve

Directions:

1. Whisk the lemon peel with honey, garlic powder, hot water, and ground pepper in a small bowl.

2. Rub this honey mixture over the salmon fillet liberally.

3. Set a suitable skillet over moderate heat and add olive oil to heat.

4. Set the spiced salmon fillets in the pan and sear them for 4 minutes per side.

5. Garnish with dill.

6. Serve warm.

Nutrition:

- Calories: 264
- Total Fat: 14.1g
- Cholesterol: 50mg
- Sodium: 55mg

- Calcium: 67mg
- Phosphorus: 147mg
- Potassium: 192mg

Meat and Poultry

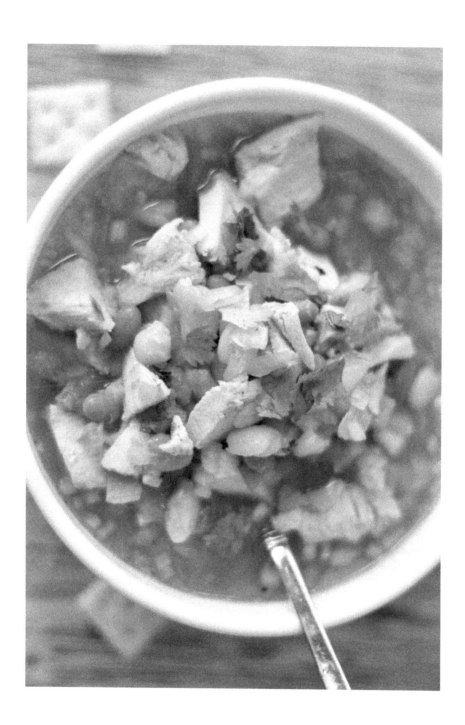

Apple Spice Pork Chops

Preparation time: 10 minutes

Cooking time: 10 minutes

Servings: 4

Ingredients:

- 2 medium apples: peeled, cored, sliced
- 1 pound pork chops
- 1/4 teaspoon salt
- 1/4 cup brown sugar
- 1/4 teaspoon ground nutmeg
- 1/4 teaspoon ground black pepper
- 1/4 teaspoon cinnamon
- 2 tablespoons unsalted butter

Directions:

1. Switch on the broiler, let it preheat, then place pork chops in it and cook for 5 minutes per side until done.

2. Meanwhile, take a medium-sized skillet pan, place it over medium heat, add butter and when it melts, add apples, sprinkle with black pepper, salt, sugar, cinnamon, and nutmeg, stir well and cook for 8 minutes, or until apples are tender and the sauce has thickened to the desired level.

3. When done, spoon the applesauce over pork chops and serve.

Nutrition:

- Calories: 306
- Fat: 16 g
- Protein: 22 g
- Carbohydrates: 21 g
- Fiber: 1.2 g
- Cholesterol: 88 ml
- Sodium: 115 mg
- Potassium: 122 mg
- Phosphorous: 144 mg

Beef Stew With Apple Cider

Preparation time: 15 minutes

Cooking time: 10 hours

Servings: 8

Ingredients:

- 1/2 cup potatoes, cubed
- 2 lb. beef cubes
- 7 tablespoons all-purpose flour, divided
- 1/4 teaspoon thyme
- Black pepper to taste
- 3 tablespoons oil
- 1/4 cup carrot, sliced
- 1 cup onion, diced
- 1/2 cup celery, diced
- 1 cup apples, diced
- 2 cups apple cider
- 1/2 cups water
- 2 tablespoons apple cider vinegar

Directions:

1. Double boil the potatoes (to reduce the amount of potassium) in a pot of water.

2. In a shallow dish, mix the half of the flour, thyme and pepper.

3. Coat all sides of beef cubes with the mixture.

4. In a pan over medium heat, add the oil and cook the beef cubes until brown. Set aside.

5. Layer the ingredients in your slow cooker.

6. Put the carrots, potatoes, onions, celery, beef and apple.

7. In a bowl, mix the cider, vinegar and 1 cup water.

8. Add this to the slow cooker.

9. Cook on low setting for 10 hours.

10. Stir in the remaining flour to thicken the soup.

Nutrition:

- Calories: 365
- Protein: 33 g
- Carbohydrates: 20 g
- Fat: 17 g
- Cholesterol: 73 mg
- Sodium: 80 mg
- Potassium: 140 mg
- Phosphorus: 144 mg
- Calcium: 36 mg
- Fiber: 2.2 g

Lamb Stew

Preparation time: 30 minutes

Cooking time: 1 hour and 40 minutes

Servings: 6

Ingredients:

- 1 lb. boneless lamb shoulder, trimmed and cubes
- Black pepper to taste
- 1/4 cup all-purpose flour
- 1 tablespoon olive oil
- 1 onion, chopped
- 3 cloves of garlic, chopped
- 1/2 cup tomato sauce
- 2 cups low-sodium beef broth
- 1 teaspoon dried thyme
- 2 parsnips, sliced
- 2 carrots, sliced
- 1 cup frozen peas

Directions:

1. Season lamb with pepper.
2. Coat evenly with flour.
3. Pour oil in a pot over medium heat.
4. Cook the lamb and then set aside.
5. Add onion to the pot.
6. Cook for 2 minutes.
7. Add garlic and sauté for 30 seconds.
8. Pour in the broth to deglaze the pot.
9. Add the tomato sauce and thyme.
10. Put the lamb back to the pot.
11. Bring to a boil and then simmer for 1 hour.
12. Add parsnips and carrots.
13. Cook for 30 minutes.
14. Add green peas and cook for 5 minutes.

Nutrition:

- Calories: 283
- Protein: 27 g
- Carbohydrates: 19 g
- Fat: 11 g
- Cholesterol: 80 mg
- Sodium: 125 mg
- Potassium: 127 mg
- Phosphorus: 147 mg
- Calcium: 56 mg
- Fiber: 3.4 g

Beef Burritos

Preparation time: 10 minutes

Cooking time: 20 minutes

Servings: 6

Ingredients:

- 1/4 cup white onion, chopped
- 1/4 cup green bell pepper, chopped
- 1-pound ground beef
- 1/4 cup tomato puree, low-sodium
- 1/4 teaspoon ground black pepper
- 1/4 teaspoon ground cumin
- 6 flour tortillas, burrito size

Directions:

1. Take a skillet pan, place it over medium heat and when hot, add beef and cook for 5 to 8 minutes until browned.
2. Drain the excess fat, then transfer the beef to a plate lined with paper towels and serve.
3. Return pan over medium heat, grease it with oil and when hot, add pepper and onion and cook for 5 minutes, or until softened.
4. Switch to low heat, return beef to the pan, season with black pepper and cumin, pour in the tomato puree, stir until mixed and cook for 5 minutes until done.
5. Distribute beef mixture evenly on top of the tortilla, roll them in burrito style by folding both ends and then serve.

Nutrition:

- Calories: 265
- Fat: 9 g
- Protein: 15 g
- Carbohydrates: 31 g
- Fiber: 1.6 g
- Cholesterol: 37 ml
- Sodium: 141 mg
- Potassium: 102 mg
- Phosphorous: 134 mg

Chicken Chili

Preparation time: 20 minutes

Cooking time: 1 hour and 15 minutes

Servings: 8

Ingredients:

- 1 tablespoon oil
- 1 cup onion, chopped
- 4 cloves of garlic, chopped
- 1 cup green pepper
- 1 cup celery, chopped
- 1 cup carrots, chopped
- 14 oz. low-sodium chicken broth
- 1 lb. chicken breast, cubed and cooked
- 1 cup low-sodium tomatoes, drained and iced
- 1 cup kidney beans, rinsed and drained
- 3/4 cup salsa

- 3 tablespoons chili powder
- 1 teaspoon ground oregano
- 4 cups white rice, cooked

Directions:

1. In a pot, pour oil and cook onion, garlic, green pepper, celery and carrots.

2. Add the broth.

3. Bring to a boil.

4. Add the rest of the ingredients except the rice.

5. Simmer for 1 hour.

6. Serve with rice.

Nutrition:

- Calories: 355
- Protein: 24 g
- Carbohydrates: 38 g
- Fat: 12 g
- Cholesterol: 59 mg
- Sodium: 148 mg
- Potassium: 153 mg
- Phosphorus: 140 mg
- Calcium: 133 mg
- Fiber: 4.7 g

Meatballs With Eggplant

Preparation time: 15 minutes

Cooking time: 60 minutes

Servings: 6

Ingredients:

- 1-pound ground beef
- 1/2 cup green bell pepper, chopped
- 2 medium eggplants, peeled and diced
- 1/2 teaspoon minced garlic
- 1 cup stewed tomatoes
- 1/2 cup white onion, diced
- 1/3 cup canola oil
- 1 teaspoon lemon and pepper seasoning, salt-free
- 1 teaspoon turmeric
- 1 teaspoon Mrs. Dash seasoning blend
- 2 cups water

Directions:

1. Take a large skillet pan, place it over medium heat, add oil in it and when hot, add garlic and green bell pepper and cook for 4 minutes until sauteed.

2. Transfer green pepper mixture to a plate, set aside until needed, then eggplant pieces into the pan and cook for 4 minutes per side until browned, and when done, transfer eggplant to a plate and set aside until needed.

3. Take a medium bowl, place beef in it, add onion, season with all the spices, stir until well combined, and then shape the mixture into 30 small meatballs.

4. Place meatballs into the pan in a single layer and cook for 3 minutes, or until browned.

5. When done, place all the meatballs in the pan, add cooked bell pepper mixture in it along with eggplant, stir in water and tomatoes and simmer for 30 minutes at low heat setting until thoroughly cooked.

6. Serve straight away.

Nutrition:

- Calories: 265
- Fat: 18 g
- Protein: 17 g
- Carbohydrates: 12 g
- Fiber: 4.6 g

- Cholesterol: 47 ml
- Potassium: 198 mg
- Sodium: 153 mg

Phosphorous: 144 mg

Pepper Steak

Preparation time: 10 minutes

Cooking time: 25 minutes

Servings: 6

Ingredients:

- 3 pounds steaks, cut into strips
- 2 cups green bell pepper, chopped
- 1 medium white onion, peeled and minced
- 1 cup carrots, sliced

- 1/2 cup celery, chopped
- 1 package brown gravy mix
- 2 tablespoons olive oil
- 1 1/4 cup water

Directions:

1. Take a large skillet pan, place it over medium-high heat, add oil and when hot, add steak strips and cook for 7 to 10 minutes, or until browned.

2. Then add all the vegetables, pour in 1/4 cup water and cook for 8 minutes until softened, covering the pan.

3. Stir in brown gravy mix, then pour in the remaining water, switch the heat to medium heat and cook for 5 minutes until the sauce has reduced to desired thickness.

4. Serve straight away.

Nutrition:

- Calories: 340
- Fat: 340 g
- Protein: 33 g
- Carbohydrates: 7 g
- Fiber: 2 g
- Cholesterol: 81 ml
- Sodium: 185 mg
- Potassium: 196 mg
- Phosphorous: 148 mg

Stuffed Peppers

Preparation time: 10 minutes

Cooking time: 1 hour and 20 minutes

Servings: 4

Ingredients:

- ¾ pound ground beef
- 1/2 cup white onion, chopped
- 4 medium green bell peppers, destemmed and cored
- 1 tablespoon dried parsley
- 1 1/2 teaspoon garlic powder
- 1 teaspoon ground black pepper
- 2 cups cooked white rice
- 3 ounces tomato sauce, unsalted

Directions:

1. Switch on the oven, then set it to 375°F and let it preheat.

2. Take a medium-sized saucepan, place it over medium heat and when hot, add beef and cook for 10 minutes, or until browned.

3. Then drain the excess fat, add remaining ingredients (except for green bell pepper), stir until combined, and simmer for 10 minutes until cooked.

4. When done, spoon the beef mixture evenly between peppers, place the peppers into a baking dish and bake for 1 hour until cooked.

5. Serve straight away.

Nutrition:

- Calories: 264
- Fat: 7 g
- Protein: 20 g
- Carbohydrates: 28 g
- Fiber: 2.7 g
- Cholesterol: 52 ml
- Sodium: 192 mg
- Potassium: 153 mg
- Phosphorous: 137 mg

Barley and Beef Stew

Preparation time: 10 minutes

Cooking time: 1 hour and 15 minutes

Servings: 6

Ingredients:

- 1-pound beef stew meat, 1 1/2 inches, cubed
- 1 cup pearl barley, soaked for 1 hour
- 1/2 cup white onion, diced
- 2 medium carrots, peeled and sliced
- 1 large stalk celery, diced
- 2 tablespoons all-purpose white flour
- 1/2 teaspoon minced garlic
- 1/4 teaspoon ground black pepper
- 1/2 teaspoon salt
- 1 teaspoon onion herb seasoning
- 2 tablespoons canola oil
- 2 bay leaves
- 8 cups of water

Directions:

1. Place beef in a plastic bag, add flour and black pepper, seal the bag and shake well until well coated.

2. Take a large pot, place it over medium heat, add oil and when hot, add coated beef and cook for 10 minutes until browned.

3. When done, transfer beef to a plate, then add celery, onion, and garlic, cook for 2 minutes, pour in water and bring the mixture to a boil.

4. Add beef into boiling mixture, then switch heat to medium level, season with salt, add bay leaf and barley to the pot, stir until mixed and cook for 1 hour until cooked through, stirring every 15 minutes.

5. When done, add carrots, stir in herb seasoning, continue cooking for 1 hour and then serve.

Nutrition:

- Calories: 246
- Fat: 8 g
- Protein: 22 g
- Carbohydrates: 21 g
- Fiber: 6.3 g
- Cholesterol: 51 ml
- Sodium: 122 mg
- Potassium: 169 mg
- Phosphorous: 147 mg

Green Chili Stew

Preparation time: 10 minutes

Cooking time: 10 hours and 10 minutes

Servings: 6

Ingredients:

- 1-pound pork chops, cubed
- 8 ounces green chilies, diced
- ¾ cup iceberg lettuce, shredded
- 1/2 cup all-purpose white flour
- 1/4 cup cilantro, chopped
- 1/2 teaspoon minced garlic
- 1 tablespoon garlic powder
- 1 teaspoon ground black pepper
- 1 tablespoon olive oil
- 6 tablespoons sour cream
- 14 ounces chicken broth, low-sodium
- 6 flour tortillas, burrito-size

Directions:

1. Place flour in a large plastic bag, add black pepper and garlic powder, then add pork cubes. Seal the bag and shake well until coated.

2. Take a large skillet pan, place it over medium heat, add oil and when hot, add pork pieces and cook for 10 minutes, or until browned.

3. Switch on the slow cooker, place pork in it, add garlic and chilies, pour in the broth, shut with the lid, and cook pork for 10 hours at low heat setting until tender.

4. When done, place ¾ cup of pork on the tortilla, then roll it like a burrito and serve with lettuce, cilantro, and sour cream.

Nutrition:

- Calories: 420
- Fat: 16 g
- Protein: 25 g
- Carbohydrates: 44 g
- Fiber: 3.2 g
- Cholesterol: 45 ml
- Sodium: 172 mg
- Potassium: 154 mg
- Phosphorous: 146 mg

Pumpkin Chili

Preparation time: 10 minutes

Cooking time: 1 hour and 15 minutes

Servings: 10

Ingredients:

- 2 pounds ground turkey
- 1 cup cooked kidney beans
- 1/2 cup white onion, chopped
- 1/2 cup green chilies, chopped
- 1/2 cup celery, chopped
- 1/2 cup carrot, sliced
- 1 1/2 teaspoon minced garlic
- 3 cups chicken broth, low-sodium
- 1 tablespoon red chili powder
- 1 teaspoon dried oregano
- 2 teaspoons cumin
- 2 bay leaves
- 2 tablespoons olive oil
- 15 ounces pumpkin puree

Directions:

1. Take a large pot, place it over medium heat, add 1 tablespoon oil in it and when hot, add carrot, celery, onion, and garlic and cook for 5 minutes until tender and when done, transfer vegetables to a plate and set aside until needed.

2. Add remaining oil into the pot, add ground turkey, and cook for 8 minutes, or until meat is no longer pink.

3. Then stir in cooked vegetables along with remaining ingredients, stir until mixed, switch to low heat, and cook for 1 hour, covering the pot.

4. When cooked, remove bay leaf from the chili, then ladle it into bowls and serve.

Nutrition:

- Calories: 168
- Fat: 5 g
- Protein: 24 g
- Carbohydrates: 7 g
- Fiber: 3.5 g
- Cholesterol: 39 ml
- Sodium: 192 mg
- Potassium: 176 mg
- Phosphorous: 107 mg

Rice-Stuffed Chicken

Preparation time: 10 minutes

Cooking time: 1 hour and 30 minutes

Servings: 6

Ingredients:

- 4 pounds whole chicken, cleaned
- 2 scallions, chopped
- 1/2 cup green bell pepper, chopped
- 1 cup pineapple pieces
- 2/3 cup white rice
- 1 teaspoon ground black pepper
- 1 tablespoon Worcestershire sauce
- 1 tablespoon olive oil

Directions:

1. Switch on the oven, then set it to 350°F and let it preheat.

2. Meanwhile, clean the whole chicken, pat dry with paper towels, and then brush well with oil.

3. Place the rice in a bowl, add scallions, bell pepper, pineapple, black pepper, oil, and Worcestershire sauce, stir until mixed, and then spoon this mixture into the cavity of the chicken.

4. Take a roasting pan, place stuffed chicken in it and bake for 1 hour and 30 minutes until the internal temperature of the chicken reaches 180° and the temperature of the rice stuffing reach 165°.

5. When done, let roasted chicken rest for 15 minutes, then spoon the rice stuffing to a serving dish, cut chicken into pieces, and serve.

Nutrition:

- Calories: 323
- Fat: 17 g
- Protein: 28 g
- Carbohydrates: 24 g
- Fiber: 0.8 g
- Cholesterol: 86 ml
- Sodium: 118 mg
- Potassium: 144 mg
- Phosphorous: 146 mg

Apple and Chicken Curry

Preparation time: 15 minutes

Cooking time: 1 hour and 10 minutes

Servings: 8

Ingredients:

- 1 medium apple: peeled, cored, chopped
- 8 skinless chicken breast
- 1 small white onion, peeled and chopped
- 1/2 teaspoon minced garlic
- 3 tablespoons all-purpose white flour
- 1/2 tablespoon dried basil
- 1/4 teaspoon ground black pepper
- 1 tablespoon curry powder
- 3 tablespoons unsalted butter
- 1 cup chicken broth, low-sodium
- 1 cup rice milk, unenriched

Directions:

1. Switch on the oven, then set it to 350°F and let it preheat.

2. Take a 9-by-13-inch baking dish, grease it with oil, place chicken in it in a single layer. Sprinkle with black pepper and set aside until required.

3. Take a medium-sized saucepan, place it over medium heat, add butter and when it melts, add onion and apple and cook for 5 minutes, or until tender.

4. Season with garlic, basil and curry powder, cook for 1 minute until sauté, and then stir in flour, continue cooking for 1 minute.

5. Pour in milk and broth, stir until combined, remove the pan from heat, pour this sauce over chicken, and then bake for 60 minutes until thoroughly cooked.

6. Serve straight away.

Nutrition:

- Calories: 232
- Fat: 8 g
- Protein: 29 g
- Carbohydrates: 11 g
- Fiber: 1.2 g
- Cholesterol: 85 ml
- Sodium: 118 mg
- Potassium: 128 mg
- Phosphorous: 80 mg

Chicken With Garlic Sauce

Preparation time: 10 minutes

Cooking time: 30 minutes

Servings: 8

Ingredients:

- 8 skinless chicken breasts
- 1 medium head garlic, peeled and sliced
- 1/2 teaspoon ground black pepper
- 1 tablespoon rosemary leaves, chopped
- 1/2 cup balsamic vinegar
- 2 tablespoons olive oil
- 1/2 cup white wine
- 2 cups chicken broth, low-sodium

Directions:

1. Take a 9-by-13 inches baking dish, add rosemary, wine, and vinegar, pour in the broth, stir until mixed, add chicken, toss it well and let it marinate for a minimum of 4 hours.

2. Then take a large sauté pan, place it over medium-high heat, add oil and when hot, add sliced garlic and cook for 4 minutes, or until golden.

3. Transfer garlic to a plate, set aside until needed, switch to high heat, add marinated chicken in it, sprinkle with black pepper, and cook for 1 minute per side until golden.

4. Then switch to medium heat, pour marinade over the chicken, add garlic and simmer the chicken for 15 minutes until cooked, turning halfway.

5. When done, transfer chicken to a dish, switch to high heat, and bring the sauce to a boil, then switch heat to medium-high and simmer the liquid until thickened.

6. Drizzle liquid over chicken and then serve.

Nutrition:

- Calories: 210
- Fat: 7 g
- Protein: 28 g
- Carbohydrates: 4 g
- Fiber: 0.2 g
- Cholesterol: 70 ml
- Potassium: 120 mg
- Sodium: 85 mg
- Phosphorous: 85 mg

Chicken Pot Pie

Preparation time: 10 minutes

Cooking time: 1 hour and 15 minutes

Servings: 8

Ingredients:

- 12-ounce farfalle pasta
- 1 1/2 cup carrots, sliced
- 2 pounds skinless chicken breasts
- 1 cup celery, diced
- 2 cups potatoes, diced
- 1 cup white onion, diced
- 12 cups water
- 1/4 teaspoon ground black pepper
- 1/2 teaspoon dried thyme
- 2 tablespoons parsley, chopped

Directions:

1. Take a large saucepan, place it over medium-high heat, add chicken, stir in all the seasoning, pour in water, bring it to a boil, then switch to medium-low heat and simmer for 45 minutes.

2. Meanwhile, take a large pot, place it over medium-high heat, place potatoes in it, pour in water to cover the potatoes, and bring it to a boil.

3. Then drain the water, cover potatoes with fresh water, bring it to a boil, and continue cooking for 10 minutes. When done, drain the potatoes and set aside until required.

4. When the chicken has cooked, remove the pan from heat, then remove the chicken from it and set aside until required.

5. Remove fat from the broth by skimming it, then place the pan over medium-high heat, add carrot, onion, and celery, bring it to a boil, and then cook for 5 minutes.

6. Add potatoes and pasta, stir in parsley, and boil for 14 minutes, or until pasta is tender.

7. Cut the chicken into bite-sized pieces, add into the pan, stir and cook until thoroughly heated.

8. Serve straight away.

Nutrition:

- Calories: 335
- Fat: 4 g
- Protein: 32 g
- Carbohydrates: 42 g
- Fiber: 3.3 g
- Cholesterol: 70 ml
- Sodium: 118 mg
- Potassium: 121 mg
- Phosphorous: 108 mg

Chicken With Mushroom Sauce

Preparation time: 10 minutes

Cooking time: 55 minutes

Servings: 4

Ingredients:

- 1 1/4 pound skinless chicken breast
- 1 cup mushrooms, sliced
- 2 bulbs garlic
- 1/2 teaspoon salt
- 1/2 teaspoon dried thyme
- 1/4 teaspoon ground black pepper
- 1/2 cup all-purpose white flour
- 1/4 cup butter, unsalted
- 2 teaspoons olive oil
- 1/2 cup oats milk, unsweetened
- 1 1/2 cups chicken broth, low-sodium

Directions:

1. Switch on the oven, then set it to 350°F and let it preheat.

2. Cut the top from each bulb of garlic, place bulb on a large piece of foil, cut-side up, drizzle with oil, wrap bulbs tightly, and then bake for 45 minutes, or until tender.

3. Meanwhile, wrap each chicken breast in a plastic wrap, and then pound with a meat mallet until 1/4-inch thick.

4. Place flour in a shallow dish, stir in salt, thyme, and black pepper until combined, reserve 3 tablespoons of this mixture, and use the remaining mixture to coat the chicken.

5. Then take a large skillet pan, place it over medium-high heat, add 2 tablespoons butter and when it melts, add chicken and cook for 8 minutes until the internal temperature of the chicken reaches 165°F, flipping halfway, and when done, transfer chicken to a plate, cover with foil to keep it warm, and set aside until needed.

6. When the garlic has baked, cool garlic bulbs for 10 minutes, then gently squeeze the cloves, chop the garlic, and set aside until required.

7. Add remaining butter in a skillet pan and when it melts, add mushrooms and cook for 5 minutes, or until golden-brown.

8. Sprinkle the reserved flour mixture over mushrooms, stir, cook for 2 minutes, add garlic, pour in milk and broth, stir until well combined, and bring the mixture to a boil.

9. Switch to low heat, simmer the mushroom sauce for 3 minutes until the sauce has thickened slightly, add chicken, toss until well coated with the sauce, and cook for 2 minutes until hot.

10. Serve straight away.

Nutrition:

- Calories: 388
- Fat: 19 g
- Protein: 35 g
- Carbohydrates: 20 g
- Fiber: 1 g

- Cholesterol: 112 ml
- Sodium: 159 mg
- Potassium: 186 mg
- Phosphorous: 149 mg

Chicken in Herb Sauce

Preparation time: 10 minutes

Cooking time: 33 minutes

Servings: 2

Ingredients:

- 2 skinless chicken breasts
- 1/2 teaspoon garlic powder
- 1/4 teaspoon celery salt
- 1/4 teaspoon ground black pepper
- 1/2 teaspoon paprika

- 1/4 teaspoon celery seeds
- 1/2 teaspoon mustard powder
- 3 tablespoons lemon juice
- 2 tablespoons butter, unsalted
- 1 tablespoon parmesan cheese, grated

Directions:

1. Switch on the oven, then set it to 350°F and let it preheat.

2. Meanwhile, take a small saucepan, place it over medium heat, add butter and when it melts, add all the ingredients (except for chicken and cheese), stir until mixed, and cook the sauce for 1 minute until hot.

3. Remove pan from heat, and then stir in cheese until it melts.

4. Take a baking dish, place chicken breasts in it, cover with prepared sauce, turn the chicken to coat it in the sauce, and then bake for 30 minutes until the chicken is thoroughly cooked.

5. Serve straight away.

Nutrition:

- Calories: 272
- Fat: 16 g
- Protein: 28 g
- Carbohydrates: 3 g
- Fiber: 0.5 g

- Cholesterol: 107 ml
- Sodium: 152 mg
- Potassium: 79 mg
- Phosphorous: 31 mg

Mexican Chicken Pizza

Preparation time: 10 minutes

Cooking time: 12 minutes

Servings: 4

Ingredients:

- 2 cups roasted chicken breast, diced
- 1/2 cup red bell peppers, diced
- 1 cup kernel corn, salt-free
- 1/4 cup onion, diced
- 2 tablespoons lime juice
- 4 teaspoons chopped cilantro
- 1/2 teaspoon minced garlic
- 1/2 cup shredded Monterey Jack cheese
- 4 flour tortillas, each about 6 inches

Directions:

1. Switch on the oven, then set it to 350°F and let it preheat.

2. Then, place tortillas onto a greased baking sheet and bake for 10 minutes until its edges are light brown.

3. Meanwhile, take a large skillet pan, place it over medium-high heat, grease it with oil and when hot, add corn and cook for 1 minute until corn is lightly charred.

4. Add chicken, onion, red peppers and garlic, cook for 2 minutes until hot, remove the pan from heat and then stir in lime juice until mixed.

5. When tortillas have baked, place ¾ cup of the chicken mixture on top of each tortilla, then top with 2 tablespoons of cheese and continue baking for 2 minutes, or until cheese has melted.

6. When done, sprinkle cilantro over pizza and serve.

Nutrition:

- Calories: 309
- Fat: 9 g
- Protein: 26 g
- Carbohydrates: 31 g
- Fiber: 2.1 g
- Cholesterol: 59 ml
- Sodium: 153 mg
- Potassium: 129 mg
- Phosphorous: 144 mg

Vegetables and Salads

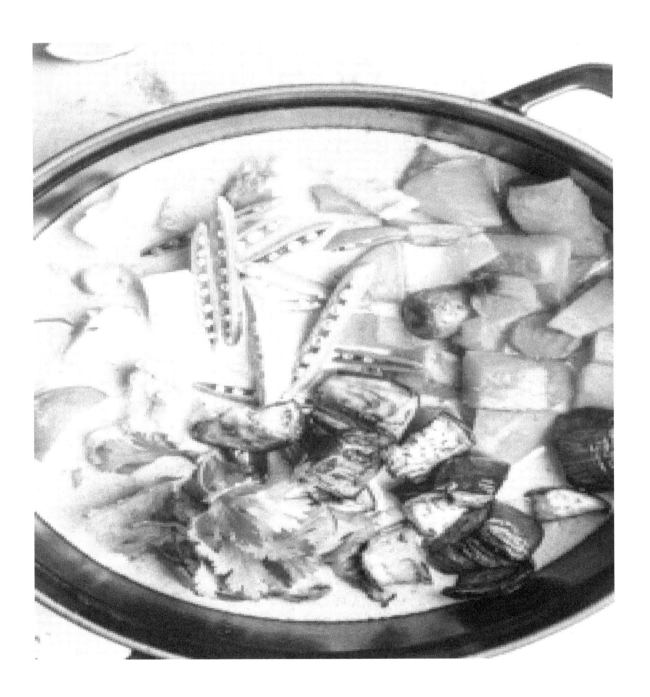

Creamy Veggie Casserole

Preparation time: 25 minutes

Cooking time: 35 minutes

Servings: 4

Ingredients:

- 1/3 cup extra-virgin olive oil, divided
- 1 onion, chopped
- 2 tablespoons flour
- 3 cups low-sodium vegetable broth
- 3 cups frozen California blend vegetables
- 1 cup crushed crisp rice cereal

Directions:

1. Preheat the oven to 375°F.

2. Next is heat 2 tablespoons of olive oil in a large skillet over medium heat. Add the onion and cook for 3 to 4 minutes, stirring, until the onion is tender.

3. Add the flour and stir for 2 minutes.

4. Add the broth to the saucepan, stirring for 3 to 4 minutes, or until the sauce starts to thicken.

5. Add the vegetables to the saucepan. Simmer and cook until vegetables are tender (for six to eight minutes).

6. When the vegetables are done, pour the mixture into a 3-quart casserole dish.

7. Sprinkle the vegetables with the crushed cereal.

8. Bake for 20 to 25 minutes or until the cereal is golden brown and the filling is bubbling. Let cool for 5 minutes and serve.

Nutrition:

- Calories: 234
- Total fat: 18g
- Saturated fat: 3g
- Sodium: 139mg
- Phosphorus: 21mg
- Potassium: 195mg
- Carbohydrates: 16g
- Fiber: 3g
- Protein: 3g
- Sugar: 5g

Chilaquiles

Preparation time: 20 minutes

Cooking time: 20 minutes

Servings: 4

Ingredients:

- 3 (8-inch) corn tortillas, cut into strips
- 2 tablespoons extra-virgin olive oil
- 12 tomatillos, papery covering removed, chopped
- 3 tablespoons freshly squeezed lime juice
- 1/8 teaspoon salt
- 1/8 teaspoon freshly ground black pepper
- 4 large egg whites
- 2 large eggs
- 2 tablespoons water
- 1 cup shredded pepper jack cheese

Directions:

1. In a dry nonstick skillet, toast the tortilla strips over medium heat until they are crisp, tossing the pan and stirring occasionally. This should take 4 to 6 minutes. Remove the strips from the pan and set aside.

2. In the same skillet, heat the olive oil over medium heat and add the tomatillos, lime juice, salt, and pepper. Cook and frequently stir for about 8 to 10 minutes until the tomatillos start to break down and form a sauce. Transfer the sauce to a bowl and set aside.

3. In a small bowl, beat the egg whites, eggs, and water and add to the skillet. Cook the eggs for 3 to 4 minutes, occasionally stirring until they are set and cooked to 160°F.

4. Preheat the oven to 400°F.

5. Toss the tortilla strips in the tomatillo sauce and place in a casserole dish. Top with the scrambled eggs and cheese.

6. Bake for 10 to 15 minutes, or until the cheese starts to brown. Serve.

Nutrition:

- Calories: 312
- Total fat: 20g
- Saturated fat: 8g
- Sodium: 145mg
- Phosphorus: 147mg
- Potassium: 153mg
- Carbohydrates: 19g
- Fiber: 3g
- Protein: 15g
- Sugar: 5g

Spinach Alfredo Lasagna Rolls

Preparation time: 25 minutes

Cooking time: 50 minutes

Servings: 4

Ingredients:

- 4 whole-grain lasagna noodles
- 2 tablespoons extra-virgin olive oil
- 1 large onion, chopped
- 2 cups frozen whole-leaf spinach, thawed (measure while frozen)
- 1 (8-ounce) cream cheese, divided
- 1/3 cup shredded Parmesan cheese

Directions:

1. Bring a large pot of water to a boil over high heat and add the lasagna noodles. Simmer for 8 to 9 minutes or until the pasta is almost al dente but still has a thin white line in the center. Drain, reserving 1/4 cup of the pasta water, and set aside.

2. Meanwhile, in a saucepan, heat the olive oil over medium heat. Add the onions and cook for 6 to 8 minutes, stirring, until the onions are tender and starting to turn brown.

3. While the onions are cooking, drain the spinach and put the leaves into some paper towels. Squeeze well to remove most of the water from the spinach.

4. Add the spinach to the onions, stir, and turn off the heat. Add 6 ounces of cream cheese to the vegetables and stir until combined. Set aside.

5. In a small saucepan, combine the remaining 2 ounces of cream cheese with the reserved pasta water. Heat over low heat, often stirring with a wire whisk, until smooth.

6. In a 9-inch baking sheet, place 2 tablespoons of the cream cheese sauce.

7. On a work surface, place the lasagna noodles. Divide the spinach mixture among them and roll them up.

8. Place the rolls, seam-side down, on the sauce in the casserole. Top with the remaining sauce.

9. Sprinkle the lasagna rolls with Parmesan cheese. Bake for 25 to 35 minutes, or until the lasagna is bubbling and the top starts to brown.

Nutrition:

- Calories: 388
- Total fat: 24g
- Saturated fat: 7g
- Sodium: 111mg
- Phosphorus: 119mg
- Potassium: 178mg
- Carbohydrates: 34g
- Fiber: 9g
- Protein: 13g
- Sugar: 5g

Crustless Cabbage Quiche

Preparation time: 10 minutes

Cooking time: 40 minutes

Servings: 6

Ingredients:

- Olive oil cooking spray
- 2 tablespoons extra-virgin olive oil
- 3 cups coleslaw blend with carrots
- 3 large eggs, beaten
- 3 large egg whites, beaten
- 1/2 cup Half-and-Half
- 1 teaspoon dried dill weed
- 1/8 teaspoon salt
- 1/8 teaspoon freshly ground black pepper
- 1 cup grated Swiss cheese

Directions:

1. Preheat the oven to 350°F. Spray pie plate (9-inch) with cooking spray and set aside.

2. In a skillet, put oil in medium heat. Add the coleslaw mix and cook for 4 to 6 minutes, stirring, until the cabbage is tender. Transfer the vegetables from the pan to a medium bowl to cool.

3. Meanwhile, in another medium bowl, combine the eggs and egg whites, Half-and-Half, dill, salt, and pepper, and beat to combine.

4. Stir the cabbage mixture into the egg mixture and pour it into the prepared pie plate.

5. Sprinkle with the cheese.

6. Bake for 30 to 35 minutes, or until the mixture is puffed, set, and light golden brown. Let stand for 5 minutes, then slice to serve.

Nutrition:

- Calories: 203
- Total fat: 16g
- Saturated fat: 6g
- Sodium: 167mg
- Phosphorus: 169mg
- Potassium: 145mg
- Carbohydrates: 5g
- Fiber: 1g
- Protein: 11g
- Sugar: 4g

Vegetable Green Curry

Preparation time: 20 minutes

Cooking time: 20 minutes

Servings: 6

Ingredients:

- 2 tablespoons extra-virgin olive oil
- 1 head broccoli, cut into florets
- 1 bunch asparagus, cut into 2-inch lengths
- 3 tablespoons water
- 2 tablespoons green curry paste
- 1 medium eggplant
- 1/8 teaspoon salt
- 1/8 teaspoon freshly ground black pepper
- 2/3 cup plain whole-milk yogurt

Directions:

1. Put olive oil in a large saucepan on medium heat. Add the broccoli and stir-fry for 5 minutes. Add the asparagus and stir-fry for another 3 minutes.

2. Meanwhile, in a small bowl, combine the water with the green curry paste.

3. Add the eggplant, curry-water mixture, salt, and pepper. Stir-fry or until vegetables are all tender.

4. Add the yogurt. Heat through, but avoid simmering. Serve.

Nutrition:

- Calories: 113
- Total fat: 6g
- Saturated fat: 1g
- Sodium: 107mg
- Phosphorus: 117mg
- Potassium: 178mg
- Carbohydrates: 13g
- Fiber: 6g
- Protein: 5g
- Sugar: 7g

Fragrant Egg Fried Rice

Preparation time: 10 minutes

Cooking time: 20 minutes

Servings: 4

Ingredients:

- 1 stalk lemongrass
- 1 cup basmati rice
- 1 tbsp. olive oil
- 1 green onion sliced
- 1-inch piece ginger peeled, chopped fine
- 1 1/2 tsp. coriander seeds
- 1 1/2 tsp. cumin seeds
- 2 cups low-sodium vegetable stock
- 1/4 cup chopped cilantro
- 1 diced red pepper
- 1 beaten egg

Directions:

1. Finely chop the peeled lemongrass.
2. Rinse the rice in cold water and drain through a sieve.
3. Heat the oil in a large stockpot and add the lemongrass, spices, ginger, and onion.
4. Cook for 3 minutes, stirring continuously.
5. Add the rice and cook for 1 more minute, stirring frequently.
6. Add the stock and bring to a boil. Add the beaten egg.
7. Cover the pan and simmer 18 minutes or until rice is not crunchy.
8. Remove from heat and fluff with a fork.
9. Add cilantro.

Nutrition:

- Calories: 105.4
- Protein: 2.7g
- Sodium: 23.2mg
- Phosphorus: 4.5mg
- Potassium: 48.9mg

Tofu Stir Fry

Preparation time: 15 minutes

Cooking time: 20 minutes

Servings: 4

Ingredients:

- 1 teaspoon sugar
- 1 tablespoon lime juice
- 1 tablespoon low sodium soy sauce
- 2 tablespoons cornstarch
- 2 egg whites, beaten
- 1/2 cup unseasoned breadcrumbs
- 1 tablespoon vegetable oil
- 16 ounces tofu, cubed
- 1 clove of garlic, minced
- 1 tablespoon sesame oil
- 1 red bell pepper, sliced into strips
- 1 cup broccoli florets
- 1 teaspoon herb seasoning blend
- Dash black pepper
- Sesame seeds
- Steamed white rice.

Directions:

1. Dissolve sugar in a mixture of lime juice and soy sauce. Set aside.

2. In the first bowl, put the cornstarch. Add the egg whites to the second bowl. Place the breadcrumbs in the third bowl. Dip each tofu cubes in the first.

3. In the second and third bowls, pour vegetable oil into a pan over medium heat. Cook tofu cubes until golden.

4. Drain the tofu and set aside.

5. Remove the oil from the pan and add sesame oil. Add garlic, bell pepper, and broccoli.

6. Cook until crisp-tender. Season with the seasoning blend and pepper. Put the tofu back and toss to mix. Pour soy sauce mixture on top and transfer to serving bowls. Garnish with the sesame seeds and serve on top of white rice.

Nutrition:

-

Calories: 401

- Protein: 19g
- Sodium: 131mg
- Potassium: 117mg
- Phosphorus: 147mg
- Calcium: 253mg.

Broccoli Pancake

Preparation time: 10 minutes

Cooking time: 5 minutes

Servings: 4

Ingredients:

- 3 cups broccoli florets, diced
- 2 eggs, beaten
- 2 tablespoons all-purpose flour
- 1/2 cup onion, chopped
- 2 tablespoons olive oil.

Directions:

1. Boil broccoli in water for 5 minutes. Drain and set aside. Mix egg and flour. Add onion and broccoli to the mixture.

2. Cook the broccoli pancake until brown on both sides.

Nutrition:

- Calories: 140
- Protein: 6 g
- Sodium: 58mg
- Potassium: 162mg
- Phosphorus: 101mg

Carrot Casserole

Preparation time: 10 minutes

Cooking time: 20 minutes

Servings: 8

Ingredients:

- 1-pound carrots, sliced into rounds
- 12 low-sodium crackers
- 2 tablespoons butter
- 2 tablespoons onion, chopped
- 1/4 cup cheddar cheese, shredded.

Directions:

1. Preheat your oven to 350°F.
2. Boil carrots in a pot of water until tender.
3. Drain the carrots and reserve 1/4 cup liquid.
4. Mash carrots.
5. Add all the ingredients into the carrots except cheese.
6. Place the mashed carrots in a casserole dish.
7. Sprinkle cheese on top and bake in the oven for 15 minutes.

Nutrition:

- Calories: 97
- Protein: 2g
- Sodium: 174mg
- Potassium: 153mg
- Phosphorous: 19mg

Eggplant Fries

Preparation time: 10 minutes

Cooking time: 5 minutes

Servings: 6

Ingredients:

- 2 eggs, beaten
- 1 cup almond milk
- 1 teaspoon hot sauce
- 3/4 cup cornstarch
- 3 teaspoons dry ranch seasoning mix
- 3/4 cup dry breadcrumbs
- 1 eggplant, sliced into strips
- 1/2 cup oil.

Directions:

1. In a bowl, mix eggs, milk, and hot sauce.

2. In a dish, mix cornstarch, seasoning, and breadcrumbs.

3. Dip first the eggplant strips in the egg mixture.

4. Coat each strip with the cornstarch mixture.

5. Pour oil into a pan over medium heat.

6. Once hot, add the fries and cook for 3 minutes or until golden.

Nutrition:

- Calories: 234
- Protein: 7g
- Sodium: 96mg
- Potassium: 115mg
- Phosphorus: 86mg
- Calcium: 70mg

Salad With Strawberries and Goat Cheese

Preparation time: 15 minutes

Cooking time: 0 minute

Servings: 2

Ingredients:

- Baby lettuce, to taste
- 1-pint strawberries
- Balsamic vinegar
- Extra virgin olive oil
- 1/4 teaspoon black pepper
- 8-ounce soft goat cheese.

Directions:

1. Prepare the lettuce by washing and drying it, then cut the strawberries.

2. Cut the soft goat cheese into 8 pieces. Put together the balsamic vinegar and the extra virgin olive oil in a large cup with a whisk.

3. Mix the strawberries pressing them and putting them in a bowl, add the dressing and mix, divide the lettuce into four dishes, and cut the other strawberries, arranging them on the salad.

4. Put cheese slices on top and add pepper. Serve and enjoy!

Nutrition:

- Calories: 300
- Protein: 13g
- Sodium: 185mg
- Potassium: 107mg
- Phosphorus: 143mg.

Cabbage-Stuffed Mushrooms

Preparation time: 20 minutes

Cooking time: 25 minutes

Servings: 6

Ingredients:

- 6 Portobello mushrooms
- 3 tablespoons extra-virgin olive oil
- 1 onion, chopped
- 1 teaspoon minced peeled fresh ginger
- 2 cups shredded red cabbage
- 1/8 Teaspoon salt
- 1/8 Teaspoon freshly ground black pepper
- 3 tablespoons water
- 1 cup shredded Monterey Jack cheese.

Directions:

1. Rinse the mushrooms briefly and pat dry. Remove the stems and discard. Using a spoon, scrape out the dark gills on the underside of the mushroom cap. Set aside.

2. In a medium skillet, heat the olive oil over medium heat and cook the onion and ginger for 2 to 3 minutes, stirring until it is fragrant. Add the cabbage, salt, and pepper and sauté for 3 minutes, stirring frequently.

3. Add the water, cover, and steam the cabbage for 3 to 4 minutes, or until it is tender. Remove the vegetables from the skillet and place in a medium bowl; let cool for 10 minutes, then stir in the cheese. Preheat the oven to 400°F. Place the caps on a baking sheet and divide the filling among the mushrooms.

4. Bake for 15 to 17 minutes, or until the mushrooms are tender and the filling is light golden brown.

5. Serve.

Nutrition:

- Calories: 163
- Sodium: 179mg
- Phosphorus: 129mg
- Potassium: 178mg
- Protein: 7g.

Vegetarian

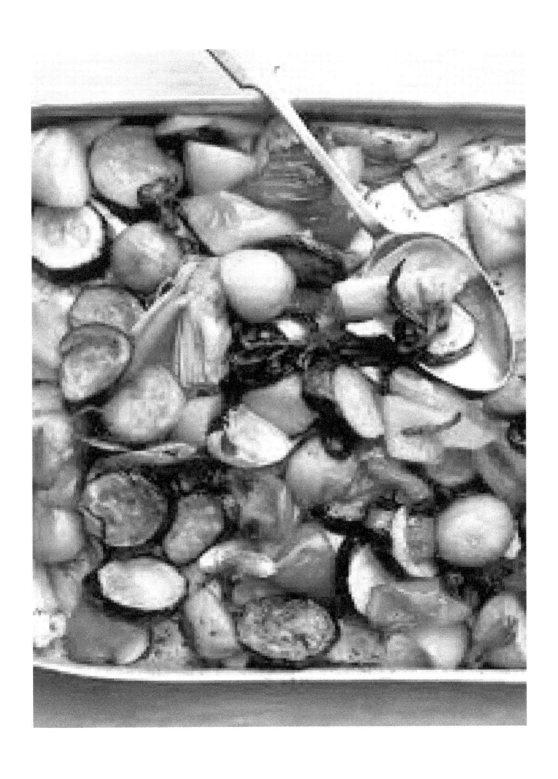

Grilled Squash

Preparation time: 10 minutes

Cooking time: 6 minutes

Servings: 8

Ingredients:

- 4 crookneck squash, rinsed, drained, and sliced
- Cooking spray
- 1/4 teaspoon garlic powder
- 1/4 teaspoon black pepper.

Directions:

1. Arrange squash on a baking sheet. Spray with oil. Season with garlic powder and pepper.

2. Grill for 3 minutes per side or until tender but not too soft.

Nutrition:

- Calories: 17
- Protein: 1g
- Sodium : 0 mg
- Potassium: 6mg
- Phosphorus: 39mg
- Calcium: 16mg
- Fiber: 1.1 g.

Thai Tofu Broth

Preparation time: 5 minutes

Cooking time: 15 minutes

Servings: 4

- 1 cup rice noodles
- 1/2 sliced onion
- 6 ounces drained, pressed, and cubed tofu
- 1/4 cup sliced scallions
- 1/2 cup water
- 1/2 cup canned water chestnuts
- 1/2 cup rice milk
- 1 tablespoon coconut oil
- 1/2 finely sliced chili
- 1 cup snow peas.

Directions:

1. Heat the oil in a wok on a high heat and then sauté the tofu until brown on each side. Add the onion and sauté for 2-3 minutes.

2. Add the rice milk and water to the wok until bubbling.

3. Lower to medium heat and add the noodles, chili, and water chestnuts.

4. Allow to simmer for 10-15 minutes, and then add the sugar snap peas for 5 minutes. Serve with a sprinkle of scallions.

Nutrition:

- Calories: 304
- Protein: 9g
- Carbs: 38g
- Fat: 13g

- Sodium: 36mg
- Potassium: 114mg
- Phosphorus: 101mg

Chili Tofu Noodles

Preparation time: 5 minutes

Cooking time: 15 minutes

Servings: 4

Ingredients:

- 1/2 diced red chili
- 2 cups rice noodles
- 1/2 juiced lime
- 6 ounces pressed and cubed silken firm tofu

- 1 teaspoon grated fresh ginger
- 1 tablespoon coconut oil
- 1 cup green beans
- 1 clove of garlic, minced.

Directions:

1. Steam the green beans for 10-12 minutes or according to package directions and drain. Cook the noodles in a pot of boiling water for 10-15 minutes or according to package directions. Meanwhile, heat a wok or skillet on high heat and add coconut oil. Now add the tofu, chili flakes, garlic, and ginger and sauté for 5-10 minutes. After doing that, drain the noodles along with the green beans and lime juice, then add it to the wok.

2. Toss to coat.

3. Serve hot!

Nutrition:

- Calories: 246
- Protein: 10g
- Carbs: 28g
- Fat: 12 g

- Sodium: 25mg
- Potassium: 126mg
- Phosphorus: 79mg.

Curried Cauliflower

Preparation time: 5 minutes

Cooking time: 20 minutes

Servings: 4

Ingredients:

- 1 teaspoon turmeric
- 1 diced onion
- 1 tablespoon chopped fresh cilantro
- 1 teaspoon cumin
- 1/2 diced chili
- 1/2 cup water
- 1 clove of garlic, minced
- 1 tablespoon coconut oil
- 1 teaspoon garam masala
- 2 cups cauliflower florets.

Directions:

1. Add the oil to a skillet on medium heat. Sauté the onion and garlic for 5 minutes until soft. Add in the cumin, turmeric, and gram masala and stir to release the aromas.

2. Now add the chili to the pan along with the cauliflower. Stir to coat. Pour in the water and reduce the heat to a simmer for 15 minutes. Garnish with cilantro to serve.

Nutrition:

- Calories: 108
- Protein: 2g
- Carbs: 11g
- Fat: 7g
- Sodium: 35mg
- Potassium: 128mg
- Phosphorus: 39mg.

Elegant Veggie Tortillas

Preparation time: 30 minutes

Cooking time: 15 minutes

Servings: 12

Ingredients:

- 11/2 cups chopped broccoli florets
- 11/2 cups chopped cauliflower florets
- 1 tablespoon water
- 2 teaspoons canola oil
- 11/2 cups chopped onion
- 1 clove of garlic, minced
- 2 tablespoons finely chopped fresh parsley
- 1 cup low-cholesterol liquid egg substitute
- Freshly ground black pepper, to taste
- 4 (6-ounce) warmed corn tortillas.

Directions:

1. In a microwaveable bowl, place broccoli, cauliflower, and water and microwave, covered for about 3-5 minutes.

2. Remove from the microwave and drain any liquid.

3. Heat oil on medium heat.

4. Add onion and sauté for about 4-5 minutes.

5. Add garlic and then sauté it for about 1 minute.

6. Stir in broccoli, cauliflower, parsley, egg substitute, and black pepper.

7. Reduce the heat and it to simmer for about 10 minutes.

8. Remove from heat and keep aside to cool slightly.

9. Place broccoli mixture over 1/4 each tortilla.

10. Fold the outside edges inward and roll up like a burrito.

11. Secure each tortilla with toothpicks to secure the filling.

12. Cut each tortilla in half and serve.

Nutrition:

- Calories: 217
- Fat: 3.3g
- Carbs: 41g
- Protein: 8.1g
- Potassium: 189mg
- Sodium: 87mg.
- Phosphorous: 91 mg

Sweet and Sour Chickpeas

Preparation time: 10 minutes

Cooking time: 12 minutes

Servings: 6

Ingredients:

- 2 tablespoons extra-virgin olive oil
- 1 onion, chopped
- 1 (14-ounce) can tropical fruit in fruit juice, strained, reserving juice
- 2 tablespoons freshly squeezed lemon juice
- 2 tablespoons cornstarch
- 2 (15-ounce) cans no-salt-added chickpeas, drained and rinsed.

Directions:

1. In a large saucepan, heat the olive oil over medium heat. Cook the onion for 4 to 5 minutes, frequently stirring, until tender.
2. In a medium bowl, whisk together the fruit juice, lemon juice, and cornstarch.
3. When the onion is tender, add the chickpeas and cook for 3 to 4 minutes, stirring until hot.
4. Add the juice mixture and cook, frequently stirring, until the liquid is thickened, about 2 minutes.
5. Add the drained fruits to the saucepan and simmer for 1 to 2 minutes or until hot. Serve.

Nutrition:

- Calories: 333
- Sodium: 15mg
- Phosphorus: 24mg
- Potassium: 117mg
- Protein: 13g.

Curried Veggie Stir-Fry

Preparation time: 20 minutes

Cooking time: 10 minutes

Servings: 6

Ingredients:

- 2 tablespoons extra-virgin olive oil
- 1 onion, chopped
- 4 cloves of garlic, minced
- 4 cups frozen stir-fry vegetables
- 1 cup canned unsweetened full-fat coconut milk
- 1 cup water
- 2 tablespoons green curry paste.

Directions:

1. In a wok or nonstick skillet, heat the olive oil over medium-high heat. Stir-fry the onion and garlic for 2 to 3 minutes, until fragrant.
2. Add the frozen stir-fry vegetables and continue to cook for 3 to 4 minutes longer, or until the vegetables are hot.
3. Meanwhile, in a small bowl, combine coconut milk, water, and curry paste. Stir until the paste dissolves.
4. Add the broth mixture to the wok and cook for another 2 to 3 minutes, or until the sauce has reduced slightly and all the vegetables are crisp-tender.
5. Serve over couscous or hot cooked rice.

Nutrition:

- Calories: 293
- Sodium: 49mg
- Phosphorus: 138mg
- Potassium: 166mg
- Protein: 7g.

Creamy Mushroom Pasta

Preparation time: 10 minutes

Cooking time: 20 minutes

Servings: 6

Ingredients:

- 12 ounces whole-grain fettuccine pasta
- 3 tablespoons extra-virgin olive oil
- 1 (8-ounce) package button mushrooms, sliced
- 3 cloves of garlic, sliced
- 1 cup heavy cream
- Pinch salt
- Freshly ground black pepper.

Directions:

1. Bring a large pot of water to a boil. Add the pasta and cook for 9 to 10 minutes, until al dente. Drain, reserving about 1/3 cup of the pasta water, and set aside. Meanwhile, in a large, heavy saucepan, heat the olive oil on medium-high heat.

2. Add the mushrooms in a single layer. Cook for 3 minutes or until the mushrooms are golden brown on one side.

3. Carefully turn the mushrooms and cook for another 2 minutes. Reduce the heat to medium and add the garlic. Sauté, stirring, for 2 minutes longer, until the garlic is fragrant.

4. Add the cream to the skillet with the mushrooms and season with salt and pepper.

5. Simmer for 3 minutes or until the mixture starts to thicken.

6. Add the drained pasta to the pan and coat using tongs. Add the reserved pasta water if necessary, to loosen the sauce. Serve.

Nutrition:

- Calories: 405
- Sodium: 42mg
- Phosphorus: 120mg
- Potassium: 128mg
- Carbohydrates: 44g
- Protein: 10g.

Simple Broccoli Stir-Fry

Preparation time: 40 minutes

Cooking time: 15 minutes

Servings: 4

Ingredients:

- 1 tablespoon olive oil
- 1 clove of garlic, minced
- 2 cups broccoli florets
- 2 tablespoons water.

Directions:

1. Heat oil on medium heat. Add garlic and then sauté for about 1 minute. Add the broccoli and stir fry for about 2 minutes.
2. Stir in water and stir fry for about 4-5 minutes. Serve warm.

Nutrition:

- Calories: 47
- Fat: 3.6g
- Carbs: 3.3g
- Protein: 1.3g
- Fiber: 1.2g
- Potassium: 147mg
- Sodium: 15mg
- Phosphorous: 16 mg

.

Braised Cabbage

Preparation time: 30 minutes

Cooking time: 15 minutes

Servings: 4

Ingredients:

- 11/2 teaspoon olive oil
- 2 cloves of garlic, minced
- 1 thinly sliced onion
- 3 cups chopped green cabbage
- 1 cup low-sodium vegetable broth
- Freshly ground black pepper, to taste.

Directions:

1. In a large skillet, heat oil on medium-high heat.

2. Add garlic and then sauté for about 1 minute.

3. Add onion and sauté for about 4-5 minutes.

4. Add cabbage and sauté for about 3-4 minutes.

5. Stir in broth and black pepper and immediately reduce the heat to low.

6. Cook, covered for about 20 minutes.

7. Serve warm.

Nutrition:

- Calories: 45
- Fat: 1.8g
- Carbs: 6.6g
- Protein: 1.1g
- Fiber: 1.9g
- Potassium: 136mg
- Sodium: 46mg.
- Phosphorous: 52 mg

Roasted Veggies Mediterranean Style

Preparation time: 5 minutes

Cooking time: 10 minutes

Servings: 2

Ingredients:

- 1/2 teaspoon freshly grated lemon zest
- 1 cup grape tomatoes
- 1 tablespoon extra-virgin olive oil
- 1 tablespoon lemon juice
- 1 teaspoon dried oregano
- 10 pitted black olives, sliced
- 12ounce broccoli crowns, trimmed and cut into bite-sized pieces
- 2 cloves of garlic, minced
- 2 teaspoons capers, rinsed.

Directions:

1. Preheat oven to 350°F and grease a baking sheet with cooking spray.

2. In a large bowl, toss together until thoroughly coated salt, garlic, oil, tomatoes and broccoli. Spread broccoli on a prepped baking sheet and bake for 8 to 10 minutes.

3. In another large bowl, mix capers, oregano, olives, lemon juice, and lemon zest. Mix in roasted vegetables and serve while still warm.

Nutrition:

- Calories: 110
- Phosphorus: 138mg
- Potassium: 145mg
- Sodium: 144mg.

Stuffed Zucchini Boats

Preparation time: 15 minutes

Cooking time: 20 minutes

Servings: 4

Ingredients:

- 2 medium zucchini
- 4 slices white bread
- 1/4 teaspoon ground sage
- 1 teaspoon onion powder
- 1/4 teaspoon dried basil
- 1 teaspoon salt-free lemon pepper
- 1 teaspoon dill weed.

Directions:

1. Preheat oven to 375 degrees F. Cut zucchini in half lengthwise. Using a spoon, scoop out seeds, forming a trench in each zucchini half. Place zucchini in a pot of boiling water, and boil for 3 to 5 minutes.

2. While zucchini is cooking, toast 2 slices of bread. Place toast and 2 uncooked pieces of bread in the food processor to make breadcrumbs. Add seasonings to breadcrumbs and mix well. Add 1/2 cup of the zucchini cooking water and blend with a fork to get the consistency of stuffing.

3. Remove zucchini from water and place in 8 x 8" baking dish, peel side down.

4. Spoon stuffing into a trench in each zucchini half.

5. Bake for 20 minutes and serve.

Nutrition:

- Calories: 42
- Sodium: 1mg
- Protein: 2g
- Potassium: 41mg
- Phosphorus: 9mg.

Roasted Broccoli and Cauliflower

Preparation time: 7 minutes

Cooking time: 23 minutes

Servings: 6

Ingredients:

- 2 cups broccoli florets
- 2 cups cauliflower florets
- 2 tablespoons olive oil
- 1 tablespoon freshly squeezed lemon juice
- 2 teaspoons Dijon mustard
- 1/4 teaspoon garlic powder
- Pinch salt
- 1/8 teaspoon freshly ground black pepper

Directions:

1. Preheat the oven to 425°F.

2. On a baking sheet with a lip, combine the broccoli and cauliflower florets in one even layer.

3. In a small bowl, combine the olive oil, lemon juice, mustard, garlic powder, salt, and pepper until well blended and drizzle the mixture over the vegetables. Toss to coat and spread the vegetables out in a single layer again.

4. Roast for 22 minutes. Serve immediately.

Nutrition:

- Calories: 63
- Sodium: 74mg
- Phosphorus: 39mg
- Potassium: 140mg
- Protein: 2g

Herbed Garlic Cauliflower Mash

Preparation time: 10 minutes

Cooking time: 20 minutes

Servings: 6

Ingredients:

- 4 cups cauliflower florets
- 4 cloves of garlic, peeled
- 4 ounces cream cheese, softened
- 1/4 cup unsweetened almond milk
- 2 tablespoons unsalted butter
- Pinch salt
- 2 tablespoons minced fresh chives
- 2 tablespoons chopped flat-leaf parsley
- 1 tablespoon fresh thyme leaves

Directions:

1. Boil water at high heat. Add the cauliflower and garlic and cook, occasionally stirring, until the cauliflower is tender, about 8 to 10 minutes.

2. Drain the cauliflower and garlic into a colander in the sink and shake the colander well to remove excess water.

3. Using a paper towel, blot the vegetables to remove any remaining water. Return the florets to the pot and place over low heat for 1 minute to remove as much water as possible.

4. Mash the florets and garlic with a potato masher until smooth.

5. Beat in the cream cheese, almond milk, butter, salt, chives, parsley, and thyme with a spoon. Serve.

Nutrition:

- Calories: 124
- Sodium: 115mg
- Phosphorus: 59mg
- Potassium: 158mg
- Protein: 3g

Sautéed Spicy Cabbage

Preparation time: 15 minutes

Cooking time: 5 minutes

Servings: 6

Ingredients:

- 3 tablespoons olive oil
- 3 cups chopped green cabbage
- 3 cups chopped red cabbage
- 2 cloves of garlic, minced
- 1/8 teaspoon cayenne pepper
- Pinch salt

Directions:

1. Cook olive oil in a large skillet over medium heat.

2. Stir in red and green cabbage and the garlic; sauté until the leaves wilt and are tender, about 4 to 5 minutes.

3. Sprinkle the vegetables with the cayenne pepper and salt, toss, and serve.

Nutrition:

- Calories: 86
- Sodium: 46mg
- Phosphorus: 27mg
- Potassium: 189mg
- Protein: 1g

Fragrant Thai-Style Eggplant

Preparation time: 10 minutes

Cooking time: 20 minutes

Servings: 6

Ingredients:

- 1 eggplant, cut into 1/2-inch slices
- 1/4 teaspoon salt
- 1 tablespoon extra-virgin olive oil
- 1 tablespoon peeled and grated fresh ginger root
- 1 clove of garlic, minced
- 2 tablespoons freshly squeezed lime juice
- 1 tablespoon water
- 2 tablespoons chopped fresh basil

Directions:

1. Preheat the oven to 400°F.

2. On a baking sheet with a lip, arrange the eggplant slices and sprinkle evenly with the salt. Drizzle with the olive oil.

3. Bake the eggplant for 10 minutes, then remove the baking sheet from the oven and turn the slices over. Return the baking sheet to the oven and bake for 10 to 15 minutes longer or until the eggplant is tender.

4. Meanwhile, stir together the ginger, garlic, lime juice, water, and basil in a small bowl until well mixed.

5. Situate the eggplant on a serving plate and drizzle with the ginger mixture. Serve warm or cool.

Nutrition:

- Calories: 52
- Sodium: 101mg
- Phosphorus: 30mg
- Potassium: 180mg
- Protein: 1g

Roasted Asparagus With Pine Nuts

Preparation time: 10 minutes

Cooking time: 13 minutes

Servings: 4

Ingredients:

- 1-pound fresh asparagus, woody ends removed
- 1 tablespoon olive oil
- 1 tablespoon balsamic vinegar
- 3 cloves of garlic, minced
- 1/2 teaspoon dried thyme leaves
- 1/4 cup pine nuts

Directions:

1. Preheat the oven to 400°F.

2. Rinse the asparagus and arrange in a single layer on a baking sheet.

3. Blend olive oil, balsamic vinegar, garlic, and thyme until well mixed.

4. Drizzle the dressing over the asparagus and toss to coat.

5. Roast the asparagus for 10 minutes and remove the baking sheet from the oven.

6. Sprinkle the pine nuts over the asparagus and return the baking sheet to the oven. Roast for another 5 to 7 minutes or until the pine nuts are toasted and the asparagus is tender and light golden brown. Serve.

Nutrition:

- Calories: 116
- Sodium: 4mg
- Phosphorus: 112mg
- Potassium: 194mg
- Protein: 4g

Snacks

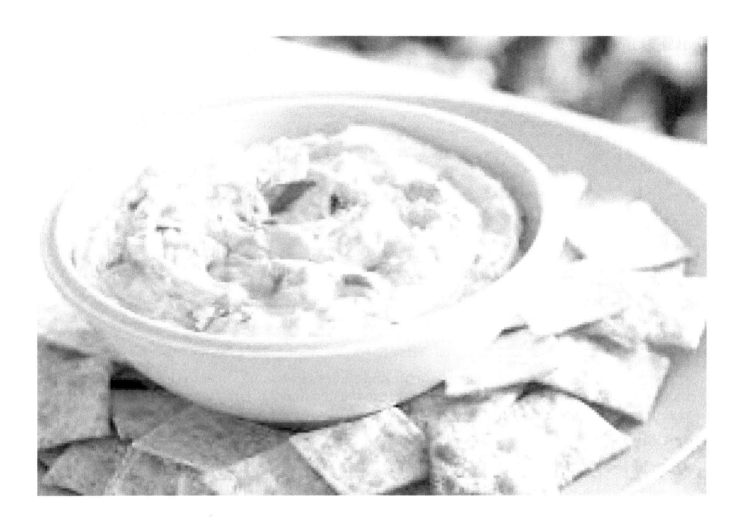

Roasted Radishes
1

Preparation time: 10 minutes

Cooking time: 20 minutes

Servings: 6

Ingredients:

- 3 bunches whole small radishes
- 3 tablespoons olive oil, divided
- 1 tablespoon freshly squeezed lemon juice
- 1 tablespoon Dijon mustard
- 1/2 teaspoon dried marjoram leaves
- 1/8 teaspoon white pepper
- Pinch salt
- 2 tablespoons chopped flat-leaf parsley

Directions:

1. Preheat the oven to 425°F. Prep a baking sheet with a lip with parchment paper and set aside.

2. Scrub the radishes, remove the stem and root, and cut each in half or thirds, depending on the size. The radishes should be similarly sized, so they cook evenly.

3. Toss the radishes and 1 tablespoon olive oil on the baking sheet to coat and arrange the radishes in a single layer.

4. Roast the radishes for 18 to 20 minutes or until they are slightly golden and tender, but still crisp on the outside.

5. While the radishes are roasting, whisk together the remaining 2 tablespoons of olive oil with the lemon juice, mustard, marjoram, pepper, and salt in a small bowl.

6. Once done, take them from the baking sheet and place them in a serving bowl. Drizzle the vegetables with the dressing and toss. Sprinkle with the parsley. Serve warm or cool.

Nutrition:

- Calories: 79
- Sodium: 123mg
- Phosphorus: 23mg
- Potassium: 21mg
- Protein: 1g

Double Corn Muffins

Preparation time: 10 minutes

Cooking time: 20 minutes

Servings: 6

Ingredients:

- ¾ cup all-purpose flour
- 1/4 cup yellow cornmeal
- 2 tablespoons brown sugar
- 1 teaspoon cream tartar
- 1/2 teaspoon baking soda
- Pinch salt
- 1 large egg
- 1/2 cup unsweetened almond milk
- 1/2 cup whole kernel corn
- 3 tablespoons unsalted butter, melted

Directions:

1. Preheat the oven to 350°F. Prep a 6-cup muffin pan with paper liners and set aside.

2. Scourge flour, cornmeal, brown sugar, cream of tartar, baking soda, and salt until well blended.

3. In a small bowl, stir together the egg, milk, corn, and melted butter.

4. Add the liquid ingredients to the dry ingredients and stir just until combined.

5. Split the batter among the prepared muffin cups, filling each about ¾ full.

6. Bake for 18 to 20 minutes or until the muffins are set and light golden brown.

7. Remove the muffins from the muffin tin and set on a wire rack to cool. Serve warm.

Nutrition:

- Calories: 165
- Sodium: 160mg
- Phosphorus: 55mg
- Potassium: 168mg
- Protein: 4g

Creamy Carrot Hummus Dip

Preparation time: 15 minutes

Cooking time: 0 minutes

Servings: 6

Ingredients:

- 1/2 cup canned no-salt-added or low-sodium chickpeas, rinsed and drained
- 1/2 (14.5-ounce) can low-sodium carrots, rinsed and drained
- 2 cloves of garlic, minced
- 3 tablespoons tahini
- Juice 1 lemon
- 2 tablespoons water
- 1/4 teaspoon ground cumin
- 2 tablespoons olive oil

Directions:

1. Combine the chickpeas, carrots, garlic, tahini, lemon juice, water, and cumin in a blender or food processor and blend until very smooth.

2. Situate hummus in a serving bowl and drizzle with the olive oil. Serve with crackers or raw vegetables, such as cucumbers, for dipping.

3. Store the hummus for up to 3 days in the refrigerator.

Nutrition:

- Calories: 116
- Sodium: 24mg
- Phosphorus: 77mg
- Potassium: 122mg
- Protein: 3g

Roasted Red Pepper Dip

Preparation time: 10 minutes

Cooking time: 0 minutes

Servings: 4

Ingredients:

- 1 (7-ounce) jar roasted red peppers, drained
- 4 ounces cream cheese, softened
- 2 tablespoons freshly squeezed lemon juice
- 2 scallions, white and green parts, chopped
- 1/8 teaspoon garlic powder

Directions:

1. Combine the peppers, cream cheese, lemon juice, scallions, and garlic powder in a blender or food processor and blend or process until smooth or desired texture is reached.

2. Serve immediately.

Nutrition:

- Calories: 124
- Sodium: 197mg
- Phosphorus: 43mg

- Potassium: 155mg
- Protein: 2g

Cheesy Rice–Stuffed Mushrooms

Preparation time: 10 minutes

Cooking time: 20 minutes

Servings: 6

Ingredients:

- 6 (3-inch-diameter) portobello mushrooms
- 1 tablespoon olive oil
- 1 small red onion, diced

- 1 cup shredded part-skim mozzarella cheese
- 1/2 cup cooked brown rice
- 1/2 teaspoon dried oregano leaves
- Pinch salt

- Pinch freshly ground black pepper

Directions:

1. Preheat the oven to 400°F.

2. Carefully remove and dice the mushroom stems. Place the mushroom heads gill side up on the baking sheet and put aside.

3. Using a small skillet over medium heat, cook olive oil.

4. Sauté the mushroom stems and onion until the vegetables are tender-crisp, 3 to 4 minutes.

5. Remove the skillet from the heat and stir in the cheese, rice, oregano, salt, and pepper until well mixed.

6. Spoon the rice mixture into the mushrooms and bake them for 15 to 20 minutes or until they are tender. Serve.

Nutrition:

- Calories: 109
- Sodium: 155mg
- Phosphorus: 90mg

- Potassium: 188mg
- Protein: 6g

Double Onion Spread

Preparation time: 10 minutes

Cooking time: 13 minutes

Servings: 6

Ingredients:

- 1 (8-ounce) package cream cheese, softened
- 3 tablespoons freshly squeezed lemon juice
- 2 small red onions, diced
- 6 scallions, white and green parts, sliced
- 1 teaspoon dried thyme leaves

Directions:

1. Incorporate cream cheese and lemon juice in a medium bowl and beat until smooth and creamy with electric hand beaters.

2. Stir in the remaining ingredients. Serve immediately or cover and chill for a few hours before serving.

3. Store this spread for up to 3 days in the refrigerator.

Nutrition:

- Calories: 148
- Sodium: 122mg
- Potassium: 117mg
- Protein: 3g
- Phosphorous: 8 mg

Crisp Seeded Crackers

Preparation time: 10 minutes

Cooking time: 20 minutes

Servings: 12

Ingredients:

- 11/2 cups whole-wheat flour
- 2 tablespoons unsalted sunflower seeds
- 2 tablespoons sesame seeds
- 1 teaspoon caraway seeds
- 1 teaspoon cream tartar
- 1/2 teaspoon baking soda
- Pinch salt
- 1/4 cup water
- 2 tablespoons olive oil
- 2 tablespoons unsalted butter, melted
- 2 tablespoons unsweetened almond milk

Directions:

1. Preheat the oven to 400°F. Line a baking sheet with parchment paper.

2. In a medium bowl, combine the flour, sunflower seeds, sesame seeds, caraway seeds, cream of tartar, baking soda, and salt and mix well.

3. In a small bowl, stir together the water, oil, butter, and milk until well blended.

4. Add the wet ingredients to the dry ingredients and mix until a dough form.

5. Spread dough out onto the parchment paper. Slice the dough into 2-inch squares. Poke each square all over with a fork.

6. Bake the crackers for 15 to 20 minutes or until they are crisp and light golden brown. Take out from the baking sheet and let cool on a wire rack.

Nutrition:

- Calories: 107
- Sodium: 68mg
- Phosphorus: 75mg
- Potassium: 117mg
- Protein: 3g

Spicy Tex-Mex Popcorn

Preparation time: 10 minutes

Cooking time: 10 minutes

Servings: 6

Ingredients:

- 12 cups air-popped popcorn (6 tablespoons unpopped)
- 3 tablespoons unsalted butter, melted
- 1 tablespoon chili powder
- 1 teaspoon ground cumin
- 1 teaspoon paprika
- 1/2 teaspoon dried oregano leaves
- 1/4 teaspoon garlic powder
- 1/8 teaspoon onion powder
- 1/8 teaspoon salt
- 1/8 teaspoon cayenne pepper

Directions:

1. Fill popped corn into a huge bowl.

2. Drizzle with the butter and toss.

3. Scourge chili powder, cumin, paprika, oregano, garlic powder, onion powder, salt, and cayenne pepper until well blended.

4. Sprinkle the popcorn with the spice mixture and toss to coat. Serve.

Nutrition:

- Calories: 120
- Sodium: 90mg
- Phosphorus: 67mg
- Potassium: 99mg
- Protein: 2g

Baby Carrot Fries

Preparation time: 10 minutes

Cooking time: 20 minutes

Servings: 6

Ingredients:

- Cooking spray
- 1 large egg
- 2 tablespoons Dijon mustard
- 1 tablespoon freshly squeezed lemon juice
- 1 cup panko breadcrumbs
- 1 (16-ounce) package baby carrots, cut in half lengthwise

Directions:

1. Preheat the oven to 425°F. Spray a rack that fits into a jelly roll pan with cooking spray and set aside.

2. In a shallow bowl, beat the egg, mustard, and lemon juice. Put the breadcrumbs on a plate.

3. Add the baby carrots to the egg mixture, tossing to coat.

4. Using a slotted spoon, transfer the carrots from the egg mixture to the breadcrumbs in batches and toss to coat the vegetables.

5. Transfer the breaded carrots to the rack on the prepared jelly roll pan and arrange the veggies in a single layer. Repeat until all the carrots are breaded.

6. Bake the carrot fries for 18 to 20 minutes or until the fries are tender and crispy. Serve.

Nutrition:

- Calories: 145
- Sodium: 91mg
- Phosphorus: 6mg
- Potassium: 125mg
- Protein: 3g

Tortilla Chips

Preparation time: 10 mins

Cooking time: 25 mins

Servings: 6

Ingredients:

- 1/4 tsp. cayenne
- 2 tbsp organic extra virgin olive oil
- 12 whole wheat grain tortillas
- 1 tbsp chili powder

Directions:

1. Spread the tortillas for the lined baking sheet, add the oil, chili powder and cayenne, toss, introduce inside the oven and bake at 350 °F for 25 mins.

2. Divide into bowls and serve as a side dish.

Nutrition:

- Calories: 199
- Fat: 3g
- Carbs: 14g
- Protein: 5g
- Sodium: 198 mg
- Potassium: 144 mg
- Phosphorous: 148 mg

Tuna Sandwich

Preparation time: 15 mins

Cooking time: 15 mins

Servings: 4

Ingredients:

- 30 g olive oil
- 1 peeled and diced medium cucumber
- 2 1/2 g pepper
- 4 whole wheat bread slices
- 85 g diced onion
- 1 can flavored tuna
- 85 g shredded spinach

Directions:

1. Grab your blender and add the spinach, tuna, onion, oil, salt and pepper in, and pulse for about 10 to 20 seconds.

2. In the meantime, toast your bread and add your diced cucumber to a bowl, which you can pour your tuna mixture in. Carefully mix and add the mixture to the bread once toasted.

3. Slice in half and serve while storing the remaining mixture in the fridge.

Nutrition:

- Calories: 302
- Carbs: 35g
- Fat: 6g
- Protein: 28g
- Potassium: 188mg
- Sodium: 122mg
- Phosphorous: 84 mg

Potatoes Croquettes

Preparation time: 15 mins

Cooking time: 20 mins

Servings: 4

Ingredients:

- 4 medium "leached" potato, cooked and peeled
- 1 tbsp. butter

- 1 tbsp. rice milk
- 1 tsp. pepper
- 1 beaten egg
- 1 cup white breadcrumbs
- 2 tbsp. canola oil

Directions:

1. Mash potatoes with milk, butter, and pepper.

2. Form cooled potatoes into balls with your hands.

3. Dip balls in beaten egg.

4. Next, roll balls in breadcrumbs.

5. Then, place balls in a hot oiled skillet and fry until golden brown.

Nutrition:

- Calories: 322
- Carbs: 75g
- Fat: 36g
- Protein: 7.6g

- Potassium: 133 mg
- Sodium: 60mg
- Phosphorous: 122 mg

Banana Breads

Preparation time: 5 mins

Cooking time: 40 mins

Servings: 2

Ingredients:

- 1 cup mashed ripe bananas
- 1/3 cups low-fat buttermilk
- 1/2 cup packed brown sugar
- 1/4 cup margarine
- 1 egg

- 2 cups sifted all-purpose flour
- 1 tsp baking powder
- 1/2 tsp baking soda
- 1/2 cup chopped pecans

Directions:

1. Preheat oven to 350°F. Lightly oil two 9x5-inch loaf pan.

2. Stir together mashed bananas and buttermilk; set aside.

3. Cream brown sugar and margarine together until light. Beat in egg. Add banana mixture; beat well.

4. Sift together flour, baking powder, baking soda, and salt; add all at once to liquid ingredients. Stir until well blended.

5. Stir in nuts and turn into prepared pan.

6. Bake for 50-55 mins or until a toothpick inserted in the center comes out clean. Cool 5 mins in pan.

7. Remove from pan and complete cooling on a wire rack before slicing.

Nutrition:

- Calories: 133
- Fat: 5.8g
- Carbs: 20g
- Protein: 5g

- Potassium: 177mg
- Sodium: 112mg
- Phosphorous: 90mg

Sides and Sauces

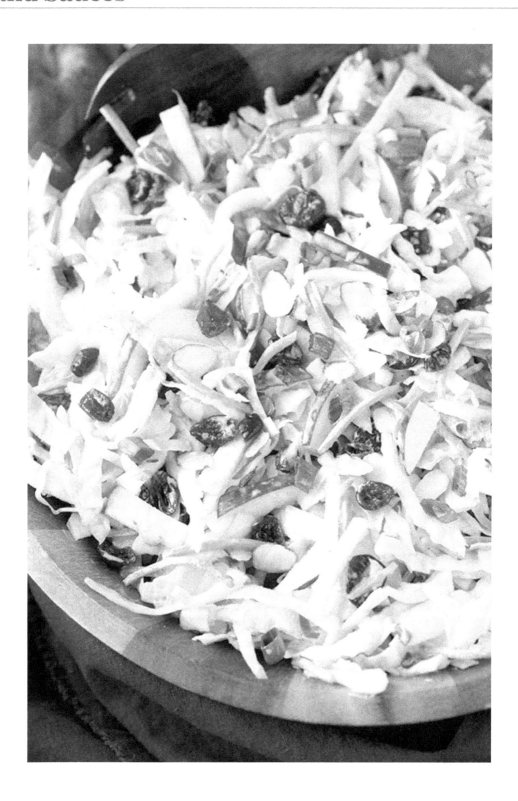

Cranberry & Apple Coleslaw

Preparation time: 15 mins

Cooking time: 10 mins

Servings: 6

Ingredients:

- 1/2 lb cabbage
- 1/2 lb shredded carrots
- 2 granny smith apples
- 2 cups fresh or dried cranberries
- 1 cup mayonnaise
- 1/4 cup apple cider vinegar
- 2 tbsp honey

Directions:

1. Shred the cabbage and carrots.

2. Core and chop the apples in small matchsticks.

3. Combine the mayonnaise, apple cider vinegar and honey in a large bowl.

4. Add the cabbage, carrots, apples and cranberries to the bowl and mix everything together.

Nutrition:

- Calories: 109
- Fat: 5.8g
- Carbs: 14g
- Protein: 1.4g
- Sodium: 144 mg
- Potassium: 100 mg
- Phosphorous: 51 mg

Baked Cream Cheese Crab Dip

Preparation time: 5 minutes

Cooking time: 30 minutes

Servings: 12

Ingredients:

- 8 ounces lump crab meat
- 8 ounces cream cheese softened
- 1/2 cup avocado mayonnaise
- 1 tablespoon lemon juice
- 1 teaspoon Worcestershire sauce
- 1/2 teaspoon garlic powder
- 1/2 teaspoon onion powder
- 1/2 teaspoon salt
- 1/4 teaspoon dry mustard
- 1/4 teaspoon black pepper

Directions:

1. Add all ingredients into a small baking dish and spread out evenly.
2. Bake at 375°F for about 25 to 30 minutes. Serve with low carb crackers or vegetables. Enjoy.

Nutrition:

- Calories: 167
- Fat: 12g
- Carbohydrates: 21g
- Fiber: 2g
- Protein: 31g
- Sodium: 188 mg
- Potassium: 120 mg
- Phosphorous: 143 mg

Seafood Jambalaya

Preparation time: 20 minutes

Cooking time: 25 minutes

Servings: 4

Ingredients:

- 1 lb wild Alaskan cod fillets
- 1 lb shrimp
- 2 cups chicken broth
- 2 red bell peppers
- 4–5 carrots
- 1 leek
- Sea salt to taste
- 1 tablespoon chili powder
- 1/2 tablespoon paprika
- 1/2 tablespoon black pepper
- 4 cloves of garlic
- 1/4 cup organic butter
- Hot sauce to taste

Directions:

1. Remove shrimp's tails and shells.
2. Slice the peppers and carrots. Dice leek, mince garlic.
3. Pat the fish and shrimp dry with a paper towel.
4. Cut the fish into medium pieces.
5. Melt butter in a large soup pot, add carrots, and stew for 4 minutes.
6. Add the bell peppers and garlic and cook for another 3–4 minutes.
7. Add all the spices and the chicken broth and bring to a boil.
8. Then add the fish and shrimp and simmer until the fish begins to flake and the shrimp turn pink and float.
9. Add the hot sauce and stir well.

Nutrition:

- Calories: 207.6
- Fat: 4.4g
- Carbs: 30.1g
- Protein: 11.6g
- Sodium: 171 mg
- Potassium: 142 mg
- Phosphorous: 91 mg

Ginger Cauliflower Rice

Preparation time: 10 minutes

Cooking time: 10 minutes

Servings: 4

Ingredients:

- 5 cups cauliflower florets
- 3 tablespoons coconut oil
- 4 ginger slices, grated
- 1 tablespoon coconut vinegar
- 3 cloves of garlic, minced
- 1 tablespoon chives, minced
- A pinch sea salt
- Black pepper to taste

Directions:

1. Put cauliflower florets in a food processor and pulse well.

2. Heat up a pan with the oil over medium-high heat, add ginger, stir and cook for 3 minutes.

3. Add cauliflower rice and garlic, stir and cook for 7 minutes.

4. Add salt, black pepper, vinegar, and chives, stir, cook for a few seconds more, divide between plates and serve.

5. Enjoy!

Nutrition:

- Calories: 125
- Fat: 10,4
- Fiber: 3,2
- Carbs: 7,9
- Protein: 2,7
- Phosphorus: 110mg
- Potassium: 117mg
- Sodium: 75mg

Golden Turmeric Sauce

Preparation time: 10 minutes

Cooking time: 15 minutes

Servings: 4

Ingredients:

- 2 tbsp. coconut oil
- 1 onion, chopped
- 2-inch piece ginger, peeled and minced
- 2 cloves of garlic, minced
- 2 cups white sweet potato, cubed
- 2 tbsp. turmeric powder
- 1/2 tsp. ginger powder
- 1/4 tsp. cinnamon powder
- 2 cups coconut milk
- Juice from 1 lemon, freshly squeezed
- 1 cup water
- 1 1/2 tsp. salt

Directions:

1. In a saucepan, heat oil at medium heat.
2. Sauté the onion, ginger, and garlic until fragrant.
3. Add in the sweet potatoes, turmeric powder, ginger powder, and cinnamon powder.
4. Pour in water and season with salt.
5. Bring to a boil for 10 minutes.
6. Once the potatoes are soft, place in a blender and pulse until smooth.
7. Return the mixture into the saucepan. Turn on the stove.
8. Add in the coconut milk and lemon juice.
9. Allow simmering for 5 minutes.
10. Store in lidded containers and put in the fridge until ready to use.

Nutrition:

- Calories: 172
- Protein: 5 g.
- Sodium: 36 mg.
- Potassium: 408 mg.
- Phosphorus: 216 mg

.

Easy Garlicky Cherry Tomato Sauce

Preparation time: 5 minutes

Cooking time: 25 minutes

Servings: 4

Ingredients:

- 1/4 cup extra virgin olive oil
- 1/4 cloves of garlic, thinly sliced
- 2 lb. organic cherry tomatoes
- 1/2 tsp. dried oregano
- 1 tsp. coconut sugar
- 1/4 cup fresh basil, chopped
- 1 tsp. salt

Directions:

1. Heat oil in a large pot over average heat.

2. Sauté the garlic for a minute until fragrant.

3. Add in the cherry tomatoes and season with salt, oregano, coconut sugar, and fresh basil.

4. Allow simmering for 25 minutes until the tomatoes are soft and become a thick sauce.

5. Place in containers and store in the fridge until ready to use.

Nutrition:

- Calories: 198
- Protein: 3 g.
- Sodium: 116 mg.
- Potassium: 115 mg.
- Phosphorus: 51 mg.

Mint Zucchini

Preparation time: 10 minutes

Cooking time: 7 minutes

Servings: 4

Ingredients:

- 2 tablespoons mint
- 2 zucchinis, halved lengthwise and then slice into half-moons
- 1 tablespoon coconut oil, melted
- 1/2 tablespoon dill, chopped
- A pinch cayenne pepper

Directions:

1. Heat up a pan with the oil over medium-high heat, add zucchinis, stir and cook for 6 minutes.

2. Add cayenne, dill and mint, stir, cook for 1 minute more, divide between plates and serve.

3. Enjoy!

Nutrition:

- Calories: 46
- Fat: 3,6
- Fiber: 1,3
- Carbs: 3,5
- Protein: 1,3

- Phosphorus: 120mg
- Potassium: 127mg
- Sodium: 75mg

Dessert

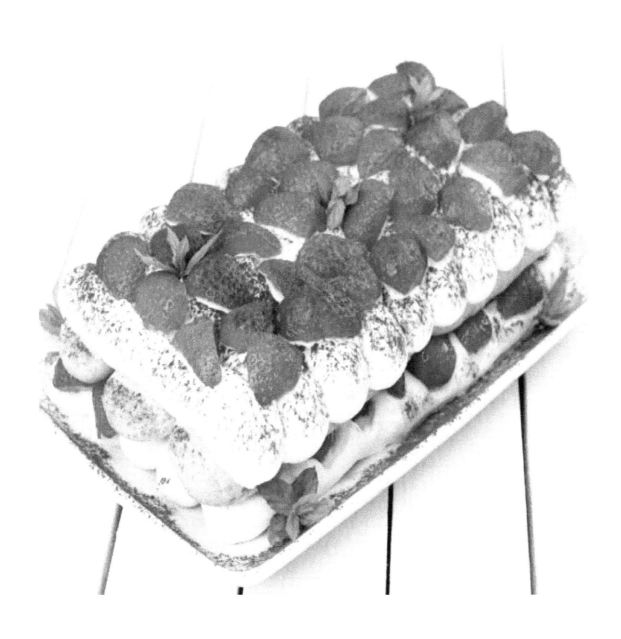

Lemon Cake

Preparation time: 2 hours

Cooking time: 30 minutes

Servings: 6

Ingredients:

- 300 g "00" flour
- 250 g sugar
- 2 whole eggs
- 100 g butter
- 2 lemons to grate (30g)
- 2 lemons, juiced
- 150 g semi-skimmed milk
- 1 sachet yeast
- 10 g pine nuts

Directions:

1. In a bowl, work the butter and sugar well and the 2 egg yolks. Then add the milk and flour (little by little), mixing well with a whisk. Finally, add the grated lemon zest, the lemon juice and mix everything until you get a homogeneous mixture.

2. Finally, add the sachet of yeast and the egg whites previously whipped. Roll out the dough into one baking dish and cover with pine nuts.

3. Put in the oven at 180 ° for about 40 minutes.

This is a high-calorie dessert, low in protein and potassium; medium-high the lipid content. Okay for patients with CKD and on dialysis. Just pay attention to the sugars, which are rapidly absorbed.

Nutrition:

- Calories: 512.7
- Protein: 9.6 g
- Lipids: 17.3 g
- Glycides: 85 g
- Calcium: 53 mg
- Sodium: 43 mg
- Potassium: 188 mg
- Phosphorus: 120 mg

Strawberry Tiramisu

Preparation time: 25- 40 minutes

Cooking time: 1 hour

Servings: 4

Ingredients:

- 4 ladyfingers
- 4 tbsp almond syrup or amaretto
- 50g sugar
- 1/2 vanilla pod
- 100g mascarpone
- 200g cream quark
- 1 tbsp chopped pistachios
- 200g strawberries

Directions:

1. Puree half of the strawberries with 1 tablespoon of sugar and the vanilla pod. Cut the remaining strawberries into small pieces. Mix the mascarpone and cream quark with the remaining sugar.

2. Break the sponge fingers into pieces and divide them into four glasses. Pour almond syrup over it, then spread the strawberry puree and strawberries on top. Pour in the quark mixture and garnish with a piece of strawberry and the pistachios.

3. Let soak in the refrigerator for an hour.

Nutrition:

- Energy: 315kcal
- Protein: 7g
- Fat: 21g
- Carbohydrates: 24g
- Dietary fiber: 2g
- Sodium: 51 mg
- Potassium: 185mg
- Phosphorous: 80 mg
- Calcium: 89mg
- Phosphate: 154mg
-

Cranberry Torte

Preparation time: 4 hours

Cooking time: 30 minutes

Servings: 8

Ingredients:

- 1/4 cup Splenda sweetener
- ¾ cup fresh cranberries
- 1 tbsp cornstarch
- ¾ cup water
- 1/4 cup white granulated sugar
- 1/4 cup chopped, unsalted pecans
- 11/2 cup graham cracker crumbs
- 1/2 cup unsalted, non-hydrogenated margarine, melted

- 1 ¾ cup Splenda sweetener
- 2 egg whites
- 11/2 cup ground fresh cranberries

- 1 tsp vanilla extract
- 1 tbsp frozen apple juice concentrate, thawed
- 2 cups Light Cool Whip topping, thawed

Directions:

1. Preheat the oven to 375 °F.

2. Combine ¾ cup of Splenda, pecans, and cracker crumbs. Add 1 tbsp margarine. Mix well.

3. Put into a spring form pan. Bake the crust for 6 minutes until browned.

4. Combine the remaining 1 cup of Splenda and berries. Let stand for 5 minutes.

5. Add vanilla, apple juice, and egg whites. Beat for 7 minutes at high speed until stiff peaks form.

6. Whip the Cool Whip into the cranberry mixture.

7. Pour the mixture into the prepared crust. Freeze for 4 hours.

8. Stir cornstarch, Splenda, and sugar together to make the glaze.

9. Stir in water and cranberries and cook until bubbly. Do not chill.

10. Place the torte on a plate. Top it with glaze.

Nutrition:

- Protein: 4g
- Carbohydrates: 46g
- Fat: 19g
- Calories: 327

- Sodium: 89 mg
- Potassium: 149 mg
- Phosphorous: 72 mg

Almond Cookies

Preparation time: 10 minutes

Cooking time: 35 minutes

Servings: 24

Ingredients:

- 1 tsp cream tartar
- 2 egg whites or 4 tbsp pasteurized egg whites

- 1/2 tsp vanilla extract
- 1/2 tsp almond extract
- 1/2 cup white sugar

Directions:

1. Preheat oven to 300°F.

2. Beat egg whites with cream of tartar.

3. Add remaining ingredients.

4. Beat until firm peaks are formed.

5. Push one teaspoon full of meringue onto a parchment-lined cookie sheet with the back of the other spoon.

6. Bake for approximately 25 minutes or until meringues are crisp.

Nutrition:

- Protein: 0.6g
- Carbohydrates: 9g
- Fat: 0g
- Calories: 37.9

Blueberry and Apple Crisp

Preparation time: 10 minutes

Cooking time: 25 minutes

Servings: 8

Ingredients:

- 4 tsp cornstarch
- 1/2 cup brown sugar
- 2 cups grated or chopped apples
- 4 cups fresh or frozen blueberries (not thawed)
- 1 tbsp lemon juice
- 1 tbsp margarine, melted
- 11/4 cups quick-cooking rolled oats
- 6 tbsp non-hydrogenated margarine, melted
- 1/4 cup unbleached all-purpose flour

Directions:

1. Preheat the oven to 350°F.

2. Combine the dry ingredients in the bowl.

3. Add butter. Stir until moistened. Set aside.

4. Combine cornstarch and brown sugar.

5. Add lemon juice and fruits. Toss.

6. Top with the crisp mixture.

7. Bake for 1 hour until golden brown.

8. Serve warm or cold.

Nutrition:

- Protein: 3.3g
- Carbohydrates: 52g
- Fat: 12g
- Calories: 318
- Sodium: 101 mg
- Potassium: 162 mg
- Phosphorous: 84 mg

Oatmeal Berry Muffins

Preparation time: 5 minutes

Cooking time: 30 minutes

Servings: 12

Ingredients:

- 1/2 cup quick-cooking oatmeal
- 1 cup unbleached all-purpose flour
- 1/2 tsp baking soda
- 2/3 cup lightly packed brown sugar
- 1/2 cup applesauce
- 2 eggs
- Zest 1 orange
- 1/4 cup canola oil
- 1 tbsp lemon juice
- Zest 1 lemon
- ¾ cup blueberries, fresh or frozen
- ¾ cup raspberries, fresh or frozen

Directions:

1. Preheat the oven to 350°F. Line 12 muffin cups.
2. Combine baking soda, brown sugar, oatmeal, and flour in a bowl. Set aside.
3. Whisk lemon juice, applesauce, and eggs in a large bowl.
4. Stir in the dry ingredients with a wooden spoon.
5. Add the berries. Stir gently.
6. Scoop into the muffin cups.
7. Bake for 21 minutes. Let cool.

Nutrition:

- Protein: 2.8g
- Carbohydrates: 28g
- Fat: 5.9g
- Calories: 173
- Sodium: 86 mg
- Potassium: 90 mg
- Phosphorous: 55 mg

Berry Fruit Salad With Yogurt

Preparation time: 10 minutes

Cooking time: 10 minutes

Servings: 8

Ingredients:

- 1/4 cup honey
- 2 cups Greek yogurt
- 1 tbsp lemon juice
- 1 cup blackberries
- 1 cup red cherries, pitted and halved
- 1 cup blueberries
- 1 cup raspberries

Directions:

1. Combine the berries with the honey in a bowl.

2. Mix the yogurt, lemon juice, and honey in a separate bowl.

3. Place yogurt cream into the center of each glass.

4. Garnish with the berry fruit salad.

Nutrition:

- Protein: 3.7g
- Carbohydrates: 27g
- Fat: 0.4g
- Calories: 117
- Sodium: 5 mg
- Potassium: 112 mg
- Phosphorous: 14 mg

Ambrosia

Preparation time: 1 hour

Cooking time: 25 minutes

Servings: 12

Ingredients:

- 1/2 cup powdered sugar
- 1 cup sour cream
- 15 ounces canned pineapple chunks
- 1/2 tsp vanilla extract
- 1-1/2 cup maraschino cherries
- 15 ounces canned sliced peaches
- 3 cups miniature marshmallows

Directions:

1. Mix vanilla, powdered sugar, and sour cream in a bowl.

2. Drain cherries, peaches, and pineapple.

3. Add marshmallows and fruits to the sour cream mixture.

4. Let chill for an hour.

5. Serve.

Nutrition:

- Protein: 1 g
- Carbohydrates: 36 g
- Fat: 4 g
- Calories: 176
- Sodium: 21 mg
- Potassium: 126 mg

Phosphorous: 21 mg

Apple Bars

Preparation time: 15 minutes

Cooking time: 50 minutes

Servings: 18

Ingredients:

- ¾ cup unsalted butter
- 2 medium apples
- 1 cup sour cream
- 1 cup granulated sugar
- 1 tsp baking soda
- 1 tsp vanilla extract
- 2 cups all-purpose flour
- 1/2 tsp salt
- 1 tsp cinnamon
- 1/2 cup brown sugar

Directions:

1. Preheat the oven to 350° F.

2. Chop and peel the apples.

3. Cream together 1/2 cup the granulated sugar and the butter.

4. Add flour, salt, baking soda, vanilla, and sour cream. Stir to mix.

5. Add apples.

6. Pour the batter into a greased 9" x 13" baking pan.

7. Put cinnamon, brown sugar, and 2 tablespoons of softened butter in a small bowl.

8. Bake for 40 minutes.

9. Let it cool and cut in 18 bars.

Nutrition:

- Protein: 2 g
- Carbohydrates: 35 g
- Fat: 11 g
- Calories: 246
- Sodium: 151 mg
- Potassium: 79 mg

- Phosphorous: 30 mg

Cream Blueberry Cones

Preparation time: 1 hour

Cooking time: 35 minutes

Servings: 6

Ingredients:

- 11/2 cup whipped topping
- 4 ounces cream cheese
- 1/4 cup blueberry jam or preserves
- 11/4 cup fresh or frozen blueberries
- 6 small ice cream cones

Directions:

1. Soften cream cheese. Put in a bowl. Beat with a mixer on high until fluffy and smooth.

2. Fold whipped topping and fruit and jam into the cream cheese.

3. Fill cones. Chill in the freezer.

4. Serve.

Nutrition:

- Protein: 3 g
- Carbohydrates: 21 g
- Fat: 9 g
- Calories: 177
- Sodium: 176 mg
- Potassium: 160 mg
- Phosphorous: 148 mg

Cupcakes

Preparation time: 10 minutes

Cooking time: 25 minutes

Servings: 33

Ingredients:

- 1 box lemon cake mix
- 1 box angel food cake mix
- 2 tbsp water

Directions:

1. Combine lemon and angel food cake mixes in a large plastic bag. Mix the two dry cake mixes when the bag is sealed.

2. Spray a small custard dish with non-stick cooking spray.

3. Measure 3 tablespoons of the dry cake mix. Place into a greased custard dish.

4. Add 2 tablespoons of water. Mix with a small fork.

5. Put in the microwave. Cook on high for 1 minute.

6. Slip cupcakes out of the custard dish. Cool for 1 minute.

7. Serve.

Nutrition:

- Protein: 1 g
- Carbohydrates: 21 g
- Fat: 1 g
- Calories: 97

Juices and Smoothies

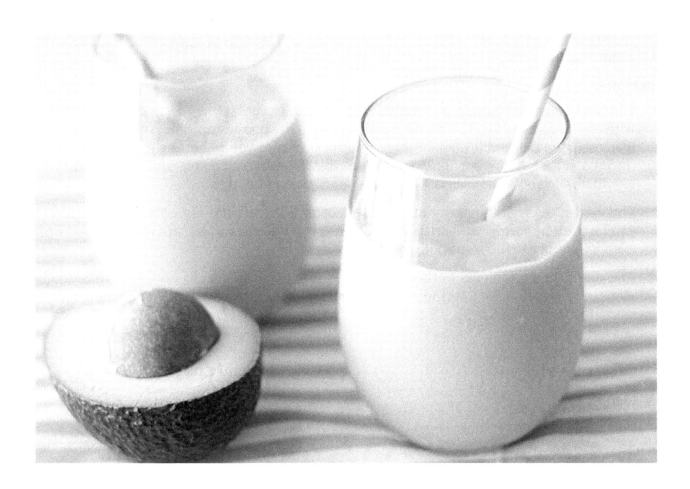

Strawberry Papaya Smoothie

Preparation time: 10 minutes

Cooking time: 0 minutes

Servings: 1

Ingredients:

- 1/2 cup strawberries
- 2 cups sliced papaya
- 2 cup coconut kefir
- 2 scoop vanilla bone broth protein powder
- 1/2 cup ice water

Directions:

1. Did you realize that papaya is incredible for digestion? The tropical organic product is stacked with compounds and cell reinforcements that help the body detox and decrease irritation. It's likewise a too delectable element for smoothies. In case you're hoping to switch your typical formula, it's a great opportunity to attempt this Strawberry Papaya Smoothie. You will need to add all the above ingredients to the blender & blend on high.

2. This beverage is without dairy and utilizes coconut kefir, a probiotic. When blended in with vanilla protein powder and crisp strawberries, you have a simple, hurried breakfast or post-exercise supper to fuel your body.

3. Add all of the ingredients to the blender and mix until the Strawberry Papaya Smoothie is pleasantly joined. I love including a crisp sprig of mint to supplement this new and fruity smoothie.

Nutrition:

- Calories: 105
- Fat: 19g
- Phosphorus: 23mg
- Potassium: 92mg
- Sodium: 24mg
- Carbohydrates: 21g
- Protein: 2.8g

Cinnamon Egg Smoothie

Preparation time: 10 minutes

Cooking time: 0 minutes

Servings: 1

Ingredients:

- 1/2 teaspoon ground cinnamon
- 1 teaspoon stevia
- 1/8 teaspoon vanilla extract
- 8 oz. egg white, pasteurized
- 3 tablespoons whipped topping

Directions:

1. Mix the stevia, egg whites, cinnamon, and vanilla in a mixer.
2. Serve with whipped topping.
3. Enjoy.

Nutrition:

- Calories: 95
- Total Fat: 1.2g
- Saturated Fat: 0.6g
- Cholesterol: 3mg
- Sodium: 120mg
- Carbohydrates: 3.1g
- Dietary Fiber: 0.3g
- Sugar: 0.8g
- Protein: 12.5g
- Calcium: 18mg
- Phosphorus: 185mg
- Potassium: 194mg.

Pineapple Sorbet Smoothie

Preparation time: 10 minutes

Cooking time: 0 minutes

Servings: 1

Ingredients:

- 3/4 cup pineapple sorbet
- 1 scoop protein powder
- 1/2 cup water
- 2 ice cubes, optional

Directions:

1. First, begin by putting everything into a blender jug.
2. Pulse it for 30 seconds until well blended.
3. Serve chilled.

Nutrition:

- Calories: 180
- Total Fat: 1g
- Saturated Fat: 0.5g
- Cholesterol: 40mg
- Sodium: 86mg
- Carbohydrates: 30.5g
- Dietary Fiber: 0g
- Sugar: 28g
- Protein: 13g
- Calcium: 9mg
- Phosphorus: 144mg
- Potassium: 111mg

Cabbage and Chia Glass

Preparation time: 10 minutes

Cooking time: 30 minutes

Servings: 1

Ingredients:

- 1/3 cup cabbage
- 1 cup cold unsweetened almond milk
- 1 tablespoon chia seeds
- 1/2 cup cherries
- 1/2 cup lettuce

Directions:

1. Add almond milk to your blender.
2. Cut cabbage and add to your blender.
3. Place chia seeds in a coffee grinder and chop to powder, then brush the powder into a blender.
4. Pit the cherries and add them to the blender.
5. Wash and dry the lettuce and chop.
6. Add to the mix.
7. Cover and blend on low followed by medium.
8. Taste the texture and serve chilled!

Nutrition:

- Calories: 409
- Phosphorus: 30mg
- Potassium: 24mg
- Sodium: 15mg
- Fat: 33g
- Carbohydrates: 8g
- Protein: 12g.

Blueberry and Kale Mix

Preparation time: 10 minutes

Cooking time: 30 minutes

Servings: 1

Ingredients:

- 1/2 cup low-fat Greek Yogurt
- 1 cup baby kale greens
- 1 pack stevia
- 1 tablespoon MCT oil
- 1/4 cup blueberries
- 1 tablespoon pepitas
- 1 tablespoon flaxseed, ground
- 1 1/2 cups water

Directions:

1. Add listed ingredients to a blender.

2. Blend until you have a smooth and creamy texture.

3. Serve chilled and enjoy!

Nutrition:

- Calories: 307
- Fat: 24g
- Phosphorus: 36mg
- Potassium: 194mg
- Sodium: 31mg
- Carbohydrates: 14g
- Protein: 9g

Blackberry-Sage Drink

Preparation time: 10 minutes

Cooking time: 0 minutes

Servings: 2

Ingredients:

- 1 cup fresh blackberries
- 4 sage leaves
- 10 cups water

Directions:

1. Add blackberries, sage leave, and 10 cups water to a blender.

2. Blend well, then strain and refrigerate to chill.

3. Serve.

Nutrition:

- Calories: 7
- Protein: 0 g
- Carbohydrates: 2 g
- Cholesterol: 0 mg
- Sodium: 7 mg
- Potassium: 26 mg
- Phosphorus: 3 mg
- Calcium: 13 mg
- Fiber: 0.7 g

Pina Colada Spicy Smoothie

Preparation time: 2 minutes

Cooking time: 5 minutes

Servings: 2

Ingredients:

- 1 cup Mascarpone Cheese, firm
- 1 cup pineapple, canned or fresh
- 1 teaspoon Stevia or another sweetener
- 1/2 cup pineapple juice, unsweetened
- Pinch red pepper flakes

Directions:

1. Mix all the ingredients in a blender. Serve.

Nutrition:

- Protein: 13.4g
- Phosphorus: 23mg
- Potassium: 55mg
- Sodium: 18mg
- Carbohydrates: 32g
- Fat: 5g
- Calories: 189

Raspberry Peach Smoothie

Preparation time: 5 minutes

Cooking time: 5 minutes

Servings: 1

Ingredients:

- 1 medium peach, sliced
- 1 cup frozen raspberries
- 1 tablespoon honey
- 1/2 cup tofu
- 1 cup unfortified almond milk

Directions:

1. Mix all the ingredients in your blender.
2. Enjoy!

Nutrition:

- Protein: 6.3g
- Phosphorus: 29mg
- Potassium: 67mg
- Sodium: 30mg
- Carbohydrates: 23g
- Fat: 3.2g
- Calories: 129.

Blueberry Smoothie

Preparation time: 5 minutes

Cooking time: 2 minutes

Servings: 1

Ingredients:

- 2 cups frozen blueberries (slightly thawed)
- 1 1/4 cup pineapple juice
- 2 teaspoon sugar or Splenda
- ¾ cup pasteurized egg whites
- 1/2 cup water

Directions:

1. Mix all the ingredients in blender, puree and serve.

Nutrition:

- Protein: 7.4g
- Phosphorus: 36mg
- Potassium: 194mg
- Sodium: 31mg
- Carbohydrates: 31.1g
- Fat: 0.75g
- Calories: 155.4

Measurements and Conversions

Volume

Imperial	Metric	Imperial	Metric
1 tbsp	15ml	1 pint	570 ml
2 fl oz	55 ml	1 1/4 pints	725 ml
3 fl oz	75 ml	1 ¾ pints	1 liter
5 fl oz (1/4 pint)	150 ml	2 pints	1.2 liters
10 fl oz (1/2 pint)	275 ml	21/2 pints	1.5 liters
		4 pints	2.25 liters

Weight

Imperial	Metric	Imperial	Metric	Imperial	Metric
1/2 oz	10 g	4 oz	110 g	10 oz	275 g
¾ oz	20 g	41/2 oz	125 g	12 oz	350 g
1 oz	25 g	5 oz	150 g	1 lb	450 g
11/2 oz	40 g	6 oz	175 g	1 lb 8 oz	700 g
2 oz	50 g	7 oz	200 g	2 lb	900 g
21/2 oz	60 g	8 oz	225 g	3 lb	1.35 kg
3 oz	75 g	9 oz	250 g		

Metric cups conversion

Cups	Imperial	Metric
1 cup flour	5oz	150g
1 cup caster or granulated sugar	8oz	225g
1 cup soft brown sugar	6oz	175g
1 cup soft butter/margarine	8oz	225g
1 cup sultanas/raisins	7oz	200g
1 cup currants	5oz	150g
1 cup ground almonds	4oz	110g
1 cup oats	4oz	110g
1 cup golden syrup/honey	12oz	350g
1 cup uncooked rice	7oz	200g
1 cup grated cheese	4oz	110g
1 stick butter	4oz	110g
1/4 cup liquid (water, milk, oil etc.)	4 tablespoons	60ml
1/2 cup liquid (water, milk, oil etc.)	1/4 pint	125ml
1 cup liquid (water, milk, oil etc.)	1/2 pint	250ml

Oven temperatures

Gas Mark	Fahrenheit	Celsius	Gas Mark	Fahrenheit	Celsius
1/4	225	110	4	350	180
1/2	250	130	5	375	190
1	275	140	6	400	200
2	300	150	7	425	220
3	325	170	8	450	230
			9	475	240

Weight

Imperial	Metric	Imperial	Metric
1/2 oz	10 g	6 oz	175 g
¾ oz	20 g	7 oz	200 g
1 oz	25 g	8 oz	225 g
11/2 oz	40 g	9 oz	250 g
2 oz	50 g	10 oz	275 g
21/2 oz	60 g	12 oz	350 g
3 oz	75 g	1 lb	450 g
4 oz	110 g	1 lb 8 oz	700 g
41/2 oz	125 g	2 lb	900 g
5 oz	150 g	3 lb	1.35 kg

Conclusion

Renal diets are specialized diets created for people with renal failure to preserve their health. As the kidney is a large organ in the body, it is vital for its proper functioning to preserve it with high-quality food rich in nutrients, which may generally taste bad but it is very beneficial if taken according to a renal diet plan.

The renal diet plan should be planned wisely so that it has all the required nutrients for the body and is less harmful to the renal system. A healthy renal diet plan can prove very helpful to the patient as he/she can lead a healthy life and can avoid certain problems.

A renal diet should be balanced so it has the correct blend of proteins, fats, and carbohydrates. These things should be taken in a specific amount. It is the amount that needs to be determined so that the diet does not harm the renal system also.

Almost all of the causes of renal failure are lifestyle diseases. Diet, hygiene, and fitness have a direct correlation to the functioning of kidneys. If we want to preserve the kidneys, we should focus on what we eat. A good renal diet consists of meals that are high in nutrition and low in cholesterol and sodium.

The diet should be maintained for a lifetime because there is no cure for renal failure. A healthy renal diet helps in the healthy functioning of kidneys, which indirectly helps to prolong the life of the patient.

Patients who have a history of kidney disease should implement a healthy renal diet lifestyle to maintain their health. The diet is to be implemented for the rest of their lives. Following are a few tips that make it easier to maintain the diet.

The diet should be based on fruits and vegetables as they are low in sodium and cholesterol. The kidneys break down protein, they lack necessary proteins, so it is best to avoid high protein food. High protein food generally consists of steak, poultry, and fish.

The healthy renal diet should consist of small amounts of dairy products, fish, and poultry. If one takes medications that affect the kidneys, then it is wisest to include a renal diet plan to be followed until the medication has completely cleared from the body.

The patient should start slowly with gradual weight reduction. You can try to eat foods that are higher in vitamins and antioxidants and lower in calories and fats. Foods such as prunes, apples, and beans possess more ingredients that make them easy to digest.

The renal diet should be taken with low sodium and saturated fats and it should contain high levels of potassium, phosphorus, and protein. It is also good to include foods rich in potassium, phosphorus, and electrolytes.

The central portion of this diet is the salt restriction method. If you follow this method, it is likely that you can improve kidney function by over 20%. Patients with renal failure may develop a renal diet plan to maintain their health and to better their lives.

It is important for people to implement a sound renal diet plan which enables them to have a longer and healthier life. It is also important to implement a healthy renal diet lifestyle that allows them to have a longer and healthier life.

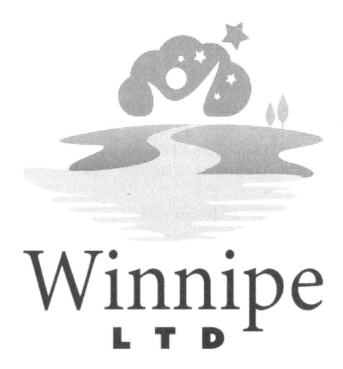

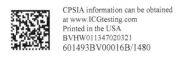

CPSIA information can be obtained
at www.ICGtesting.com
Printed in the USA
BVHW011347020321
601493BV00016B/1480